PRO-VAX

Medical Humanities: Criticism and Creativity

Vol 4

Series Editors: Maria Vaccarella, MA, PhD, Senior Lecturer in Medical Humanities, University of Bristol and Kimberly R. Myers, MA, PhD, Professor of Humanities and Medicine, Penn State College of Medicine

PETER LANG
Oxford - Berlin - Bruxelles - Chennai - Lausanne - New York

PRO-VAX

SUPPORTING VACCINES THROUGH ACTIVISM, PETITIONS, AND TRIALS

Samantha Vanderslott

PETER LANG
Oxford - Berlin - Bruxelles - Chennai - Lausanne - New York

Bibliographic information published by the Deutsche Nationalbibliothek.
The German National Library lists this publication in the German National Bibliography; detailed bibliographic data is available on the Internet at http:// dnb.d- nb.de.

A catalogue record for this book is available from the British Library.

Library of Congress Cataloging-in-Publication Data

Names: Vanderslott, Samantha, 1985- author.
Title: Pro-vax : supporting vaccines through activism, petitions, and trials / Samantha Vanderslott.
Description: Oxford ; New York : Peter Lang, 2025. | Series: Medical humanities: criticism and creativity, 2504-5229 ; vol no. 4 | Includes bibliographical references and index.
Identifiers: LCCN 2023056364 (print) | LCCN 2023056365 (ebook) | ISBN 9781800794702 (hardback) | ISBN 9781800794719 (ebook) | ISBN 9781800794726 (epub)
Subjects: LCSH: Vaccination--Public opinion. | Vaccines--Public opinion. | Vaccination--Social aspects. | Vaccines--Social aspects. | Health attitudes.
Classification: LCC RA638 .V36 2025 (print) | LCC RA638 (ebook) | DDC 615.3/72--dc23/eng/20231220
LC record available at https://lccn.loc.gov/2023056364
LC ebook record available at https://lccn.loc.gov/2023056365

Cover image: Martin O'Neill.
Cover design by Peter Lang Group AG

ISSN 2504-5229
ISBN 978-1-80079-470-2 (print)
ISBN 978-1-80079-471-9 (ePDF)
ISBN 978-1-80079-472-6 (ePub)
DOI 10.3726/b19581

Published by Peter Lang Ltd, Oxford, United Kingdom
info@peterlang.com - www.peterlang.com

This publication has been peer reviewed.

For Bary and Reuben

Contents

Images

Boxes

Abbreviations

AMR:	anti-microbial resistance
ASI:	Australian Skeptics Inc.
BCG:	Bacillus Calmette-Guérin
BMJ:	British Medical Journal
CAM:	complementary and alternative medicine
CaT:	Coalition against Typhoid
CDC:	Centers for Disease Control and Prevention
CHIM:	controlled human infection model
COVAX:	COVID-19 Vaccines Global Access
COVID-19:	2019 novel coronavirus
ECDC:	European Centre for Disease Prevention and Control
EID:	emerging infectious diseases
EMA:	European Medical Association
EPI:	Expanded Programme on Immunization
FDA:	Food and Drug Administration
Gavi:	Gavi, the Vaccine Alliance
GP:	general practitioner
HCCC:	Health Care Complaints Commission
Hib:	*Haemophilus influenzae* type B
HIV/AIDS:	human immunodeficiency virus infection/ acquired immunodeficiency syndrome
HPV:	human papillomavirus
IMD:	invasive meningococcal disease
JCVI:	Joint Committee on Vaccination and Immunisation
LMIC(s):	low- and middle-income country(s)
Men(A,B,C,W,X,Y):	meningococcal (A,B,C,W,X,Y)

MERS-CoV:	Middle East respiratory syndrome-related coronavirus
MMR:	measles, mumps, and rubella
MRC:	Medical Research Council
mRNA:	messenger ribonucleic acid
MVP:	Meningitis Vaccine Project
NHS:	National Health Service
NRVS:	Northern Rivers Vaccination Supporters
OVG:	Oxford Vaccine Group
RCT:	randomised controlled trial
SAGE:	Strategic Advisory Group of Experts
SAGE:	Scientific Advisory Group for Emergencies
SARS:	severe acute respiratory syndrome
SARS-CoV:	SARS-associated coronavirus
SAVN:	Stop the AVN
SB:	senate bill
SIIPL:	Serum Institute of India Pvt. Ltd
TB:	tuberculosis
TCV:	typhoid conjugate vaccine
TyVAC:	Typhoid Acceleration Consortium
UNICEF:	United Nations Children's Emergency Fund
UT:	union territory
VPDs:	vaccine-preventable diseases
WASH:	water, sanitation, and hygiene
WHO:	World Health Organization
XDR:	extensively drug-resistant

Preface

Vaccination is both a social activity on a grand scale and a deeply personal and individual experience. Recounting our stories of vaccination means encountering thoughts quite specific to our own lives, to particular vaccines, and to the diseases that they prevent. Add to this the understanding of vaccination in culture, the media, and others around us in society, and attitudes to vaccination can become complex. However, when considering such individual vaccination journeys, certain touchpoints may be uncovered. Many will remember being in school and waiting in an excited, nervous line to be vaccinated. My distinct memory was receiving a Bacillus Calmette-Guérin (BCG) vaccination against tuberculosis (TB) with my classmates. I asked the nurse if I was going to get a lollipop only to be told 'No, only a permanent scar' followed by a chuckle.

The BCG vaccine is now no longer given in the United Kingdom because of falling cost-effectiveness and low TB rates at the population level. While this vaccination had been a national policy from 1990 to 2005, it is now only offered for babies born into high-risk groups, such as those coming from countries where TB is endemic, including parents or grandparents born in high-risk countries. The various changing country policies for BCG have become sufficiently complicated that a map was devised to catalogue previous and ongoing policies and practices across the world.[1] One country that still is a high-risk country for TB is the Philippines. This is where my mother emigrated from in the 1970s, coming to the United Kingdom to work as a nurse in the National Health Service (NHS), On arrival she was found to have latent TB. She thus spent the first months in her new home quarantined, swallowing what she described as 'horse pills', alone in a clinically decorated room. Her time was brightened only by new friends passing a daffodil on a bamboo stick through the hospital window.

1 See <http://www.bcgatlas.org>.

Most people's next encounter with vaccination after childhood is during adolescence, when vaccines come as an option to protect against threats such as meningococcal disease and human papillomavirus (HPV). After leaving school, people also often receive vaccines before traveling abroad, for example, against typhoid and yellow fever, which have been live vaccines. Other vaccines are targeted towards specific groups of people, such as influenza and COVID-19 vaccines, which healthcare workers and vulnerable groups are encouraged to receive. However, the major point at which many are confronted with the need to vaccinate once more more frequently is for babies and children. These vaccinations are often set in national routine immunisation schedules, administered at health clinics and then at schools. Administering vaccines at this early stage offers protection before pathogens that cause disease are encountered and is why pregnant women are also recommended to receive vaccines, such as for pertussis, to pass on protection to their babies. For parents and guardians, the decision-making and responsibility for vaccination comes into the foreground, making their views and actions especially important. The majority of vaccinations on the national schedule occur during childhood, including multiple doses and boosters. Later, in older age, there are again vaccines (to protect against pneumococcal disease and shingles for example).

More sensationally, as a result of disease outbreaks, vaccines make the news and become objects of public interest: when lower uptake leads to outbreaks of so-called vaccine-preventable diseases, or of emerging or re-emerging pathogens that populations may have little protection against (and for which a vaccine may not yet exist). As experienced in recent years, vaccines take centre stage in times of crisis, being developed and administered in response to an epidemic or pandemic of a novel pathogen, such as the viruses that cause Ebola or COVID-19. Indifference, hesitancy, and even resistance to vaccination can then receive intense media coverage and become cause for government concern. However, what is notable about many vaccination touchpoints is the implicit support that is offered by vaccinating. It is something that many of us do not stop to consider. Conversely, there might be awareness for those very vocally opposed to vaccination or when vaccine policy changes, such as with the introduction of mandatory vaccination. For the majority, however, support for vaccines is often taken for granted, if considered at all.

Nevertheless, vaccination is an issue that is increasingly polarised, and with a more highly organised and influential anti-vaccine public group emerging, the need for an explicit pro-vaccine support base is becoming ever more necessary. Concurrently, the role of vaccines in society continues to change and evolve, both as a social and biomedical object. This book aims to reconsider vaccination from the perspective of those who are 'pro-vax', who actively support and vocally promote vaccines, by drawing out key episodes and features of pro-vaccine activity. I reflect on the meaning of being pro-vax and the implications for vaccination more generally. In contrast, the current literature on attitudes towards vaccination concentrates on those who are in opposition. Although this narrow view has been changing, a directed study of those who support vaccination has been lacking. That said, there have been important developments in how scholars approach vaccination as a socio-cultural phenomenon. For example, historian Gareth Millward (2019) has focused on how child immunisation became the status quo in Britain.

More generally, the public health term 'vaccine hesitancy', has currency via by the WHO Strategic Advisory Group of Experts on Immunization (SAGE), who established a Working Group on Vaccine Hesitancy and published a number of influential papers. It was further popularised by others, including anthropologist Heidi Larson who introduced the framing of 'vaccine confidence', to acknowledge a range of views that encompass delay in acceptance and not only outright refusal. I aim to further build on this work to provide value to students and scholars, as well as to a more general readership interested in topics at the intersection of health and society. Drawing on theory from the public health literature and incorporating conceptions about health from the sociology of science, this book takes a novel approach to understand how vaccines are supported by civil society. Additionally, the inclusion of images is an important aspect of vaccination communication and promotion, especially as imagery is utilised across opposing perspectives. In viewing vaccine imagery it is necessary to go beyond tropes of a needle and vial, plaster, crying child, worried parent, and healthcare worker.

I have many people to thank for helping me write this book, not least for their support and time, but also for the ongoing intellectual exchange. Laurel Plapp at Peter Lang kept me on track, the two anonymous reviewers provided incredibly helpful comments, and I have numerous peers in other countries who I appreciate for their continued academic support, particularly Jeremy Ward, Brian Martin, Heidi Larson, and Ben Kasstan. I draw heavily on collaborative work with students, research assistants, and colleagues: Alex Bowmer, Jonathan Kantor, Kate Joynes-Burgess, Katharina T. Paul, Luisa Enria, Noémi Déom, Patricia Kingori, Sally Frampton, Sarah Spellman, Shelley Lees, Tatyana Marks, Tushna Vandrevala, plus the whole COVQUAL team – Arabella Stuart, John Henry, Katherine Emary, Marcus English, Maia Patrick-Smith, Maria Moore, Naomi Douglas, Rebecca Te Water Naude, Susanne Hodgson, and Tonia Thomas.

I am lucky to have two long-term collaborators: Claas Kirchhelle, where history and sociology have combined for a journey into many things typhoid and vaccine related; and Sam Martin, who has opened the world of digital sociology to me and been a patient teacher of the lay of the land. In addition, I have an inspiring mentor in Andrew Pollard, and many other colleagues I have met through the Oxford Vaccine Group (OVG) at the University of Oxford, especially Richard Moxon, Rinn Song, Parv Aley, Seilesh Kadambari, Sean Elias, Charlie Firth, Sophia Wilkinson, Karen Ford, and Lucky Khan, as well as the continued support of Georg Hollander and Shaka Obhiozele at Oxford's Department of Paediatrics. All mentioned either very kindly read parts or discussed ideas with me, making this book the output of collective endeavour, although of course any remaining errors are mine. I am also grateful for funding from the Arts and Humanities Research Council (AHRC) and the National Institute for Health and Care Research (NIHR) to allow me to pursue this research.

Finally, my family and friends have been a core part of this journey, cheering me on and providing encouragement all the way, with a special mention to Bary, my sounding board always, and Reuben my new, little writing buddy. The previous January, I was able to expand my work on the social study of vaccination by establishing the 'Vaccines and Society Unit' hosted at OVG. I was lucky to have Katie Attwell come and join as the first visiting academic. We also very sadly lost an incredible friend and colleague last year, Nina Hallowell, who was an enthusiastic backer from the very inception of the unit. She is greatly missed by all of us.

Samantha Vanderslott

CHAPTER 1

Introduction

Controlling infectious diseases

On 13 June 1935, at the meeting of the American Medical Association in Atlantic City, physician Dr David Riesman read a paper on 'Deceased Diseases'. He proclaimed how 'the greatest triumphs have undoubtedly been achieved in the infectious diseases' (1936, p. 160). He went on to say, 'Theoretically these are all conquerable and we may hope to banish most of them in time' (ibid.). Improvements to sanitation and in standards of living (e.g. housing and nutrition) were offered as reasons for the decline in the number of infectious diseases. The sanitary revolution, which brought clean water and systems of waste disposal and hygiene, was indeed a reason for optimism. In addition, the discovery of antibiotics, used to kill bacteria, and vaccines as a preventative measure against disease are among the most important in all medicine, with both interventions having a tremendous impact on illness and deaths from infectious diseases (Armstrong, Conn, and Pinner 1999).

Antibiotics first revolutionised infectious diseases control. While mould had been known since ancient times to possess antibacterial properties, it was the 1930s that produced the sulfa antimicrobials, arsphenamine (Salvarsan), and the sulphonamides, which were not biological (Mohr 2016a). Biological antibiotic research was pioneered by René Dubos, a French microbiologist. In 1939, Dubos discovered gramicidin, the first clinically tested antibacterial agent that inhibits the growth of gram-positive bacteria[1] (Van Epps 2006). The effect of this discovery was

1 Gram-positive bacteria are easier to kill and develop resistance slower than gram-negative bacteria (Tavares et al. 2020).

to revive the stalled interest in penicillin, which had proved difficult to purify and produce in volume (ibid.). Hailed as the miracle drug, penicillin was discovered in 1928 by Scottish physician and microbiologist Sir Alexander Fleming, but took many years to be widely used.[2] During World War II, penicillin was heavily deployed to treat Allied troops, and even at this early stage, Fleming warned that overuse and misuse could lead to resistant bacteria. Following World War II came a 'golden age of natural product antibiotic discovery' (Hutchings, Truman, and Wilkinson 2019, p. 72).[3] In 1944, streptomycin, the world's first broad-spectrum effective antibiotic (Image 1.1), was discovered by Schatz, Bugie, and Waksman, and used to cure tuberculosis, tuberculous meningitis, and other infections (Mohr 2016a). In 1946, penicillin became available for public use in the United Kingdom (following use during World War II), and antibiotics were soon introduced on a large scale from the 1950s onwards to treat bacterial infections (ibid.) (Image 1.2).

Vaccination became more widespread due to the increased understanding of disease through germ theory (that disease is caused by microorganisms). The different impact that vaccines had on infectious disease in comparison to antibiotics as a preventative health intervention was that they can be deployed on a mass scale to immunise whole populations.[4] Vaccination also has a long history, and again it took time to reach the era of mass immunisation against different diseases. Edward Jenner conducted the first scientific investigations of smallpox prevention in the late

2 The 'Penicillin Project' team of scientists in Oxford, comprising of Howard Florey, Ernst Chain and others achieved a successful mice experiment in 1940 and then six women, known as the 'Penicillin Girls' (Ruth Callow, Claire Inayat, Betty Cooke, Peggy Gardner, Megan Lancaster, and Patricia McKegney), used fermenting broth to 'farm' precious milligrams of penicillin for the first human trial in 1941 (Swain 2017). That year, Florey took penicillin to the Department of Agriculture's research laboratory in the United States to scale up production, the lab added corn-steep liquor to the mould broth, and lab assistant Mary Hunt found mould that produced six times more penicillin than Fleming's original strain using a rotting cantaloupe melon at a local market (Bennett and Chung 2001).

3 By the 1930s, the first commercially available antibacterial Prontosil was developed by Paul Gerhard Domagk, a German physician (Mohr 2016b).

4 In this book I follow the CDC (n.d.) definition: 'Vaccination: The act of introducing a vaccine into the body to produce protection from a specific disease. Immunization: A process by which a person becomes protected against a disease through vaccination.' However, note that the two terms are closely related and often used interchangeably.

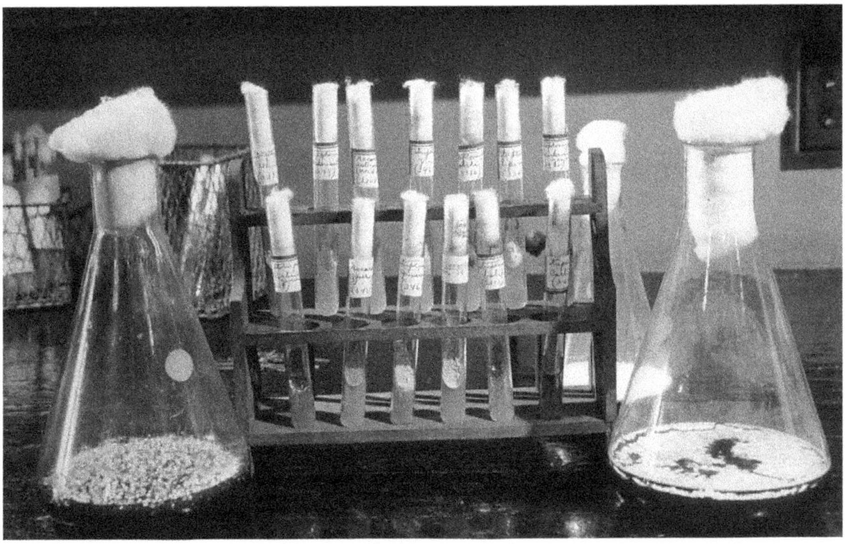

Image 1.1 Test tubes and flasks of streptomycin in Waksman Laboratory.

G. Terry Sharrer, National Museum of American History. Unknown photographer, Public domain, via Wikimedia Commons. <https://commons.wikimedia.org/wiki/File:Waksman_laboratory.jpg>

1700s, eventually producing an early version of a smallpox vaccine in 1796 (Hilleman 2000). It was then the French scientist Louis Pasteur who first successfully extended the vaccination principle to diseases beyond smallpox. In 1880, Pasteur discovered the principle of attenuation after injecting laboratory animals with a culture of chicken cholera that had accidentally been exposed to air, which led to the development of attenuated vaccines against sheep anthrax and human rabies (Hajj Hussein et al. 2015).[5]

By the early 1900s, bacterial culture techniques had yielded the Pasteurian and Kochian vaccines (chicken cholera, cholera, and typhoid from the 1870s onwards) and allowed for the development of bacterial toxoid vaccines for diphtheria and tetanus, as well as the whole-cell vaccine for

5 This experiment was part of a programme of laboratory research by the physician Emile Roux.

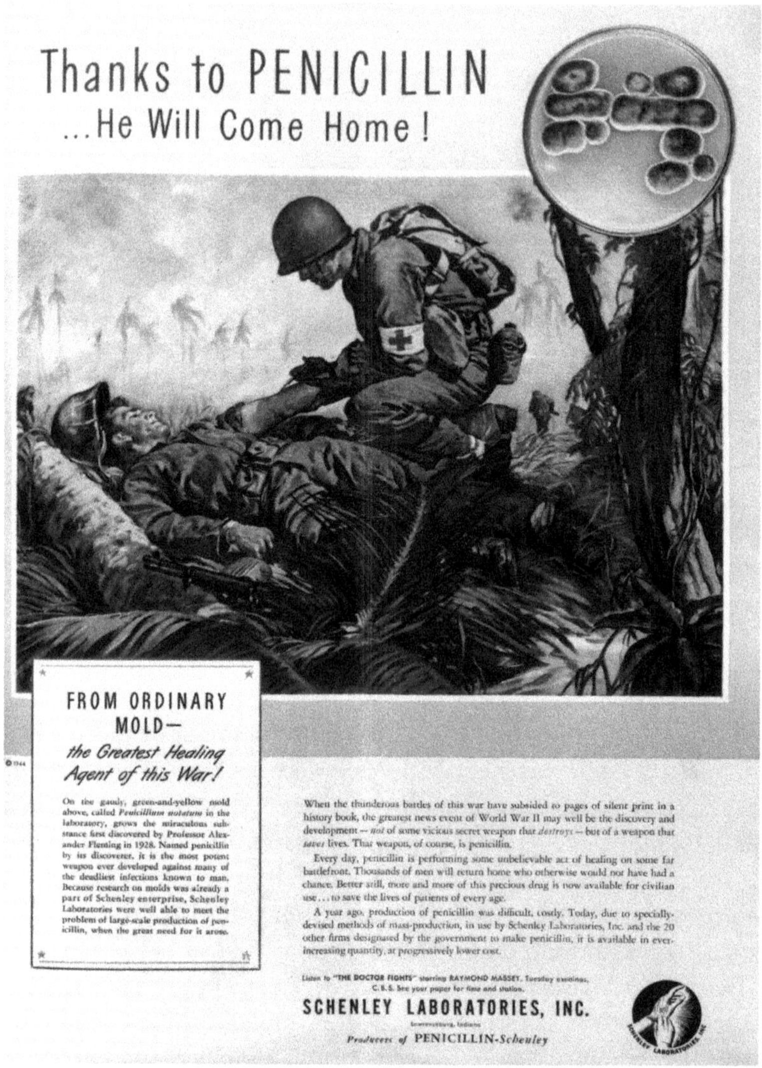
Thanks to PENICILLIN
...He Will Come Home!
FROM ORDINARY MOLD—
the Greatest Healing Agent of this War!
On the gaudy, green-and-yellow mold above, called *Penicillium notatum* in the laboratory, grows the miraculous substance first discovered by Professor Alexander Fleming in 1928. Named penicillin by its discoverer, it is the most potent weapon ever developed against many of the deadliest infections known to man. Because research on molds was already a part of Schenley enterprise, Schenley Laboratories were well able to meet the problem of large-scale production of penicillin, when the great need for it arose.
When the thunderous battles of this war have subsided to pages of silent print in a history book, the greatest news event of World War II may well be the discovery and development – *not* of some vicious secret weapon that *destroys* – but of a weapon that *saves* lives. That weapon, of course, is penicillin.
Every day, penicillin is performing some unbelievable act of healing on some far battlefront. Thousands of men will return home who otherwise would not have had a chance. Better still, more and more of this precious drug is now available for civilian use . . . to save the lives of patients of every age.
A year ago, production of penicillin was difficult, costly. Today, due to specially-devised methods of mass-production, in use by Schenley Laboratories, Inc. and the 20 other firms designated by the government to make penicillin, it is available in ever-increasing quantity, at progressively lower cost.
Listen to "THE DOCTOR FIGHTS" starring RAYMOND MASSEY, Tuesday evenings, C.B.S. See your paper for time and station.
SCHENLEY LABORATORIES, INC.
Producers of PENICILLIN-Schenley
SCHENLEY LABORATORIES INC

Image 1.2 Advertisement for penicillin production by Schenley Laboratories Inc. from *Life* magazine.

August 14 1944. Science Museum, London. Attribution 4.0 International (CC BY 4.0). <https://collection.sciencemuseumgroup.org.uk/documents/aa110070387/issue-of-life-magazine-containing-advertisement-p-97-entitled-thanks-to-penicillin-he-will-come-home-advertising-the-large-scale-production-of-penicillin-by-schenley-laboratories-inc>

pertussis. In 1921, the French bacteriologist Albert Calmette and veterinarian Camille Guérin developed the Bacillus Calmette-Guérin (BCG) vaccine against tuberculosis.[6] However, it was not until the middle of the century that vaccines for many viral infectious diseases were developed, resulting from a combination of political-economic (Baker and Katz 2004) and scientific developments (Blume, Holmberg, and Greenough 2017). A drive for collaboration between universities, governments, and private companies had been prompted by World Wars I and II for a joint effort in scientific progress to benefit human health, although this benefit was not always equitable (ibid.). Primary beneficiaries were high-income populations and companies making substantial profits. Before 1950, there were few successful viral vaccines, with the exceptions of vaccines for yellow fever and influenza, grown in embryonated chicken eggs (Hilleman 2000). The modern era of vaccinology is typically said to have begun in the 1950s, as viral tissue culture techniques further allowed for the development of many vaccines against viruses such as polio, measles, mumps, rubella, and varicella (chickenpox) (ibid.). The 1941 development of tissue culture by American virologists John Enders, Thomas Weller, and Frederick Robbins at the Children's Medical Centre in Boston, was a pivotal step in providing a medium that made it possible to propagate and manipulate viruses and so develop vaccines against viral diseases (Baker and Katz 2004).

The 1970s then marked a particular turning point to confirm earlier predictions, where through the impact of antibiotics and vaccines on human and animal health, infectious diseases appeared conquered and relegated to the past – at least for the so-called developed world (Washer 2010). In 1980, after a concerted vaccination campaign, the World Health Assembly declared smallpox eradicated (Image 1.3), as there were no more cases of naturally occurring infection (Bhattacharya and D'Avila Pereira Campani 2020). Smallpox was the first infectious disease to be eradicated, followed by rinderpest in 2011. Other diseases such as polio looked soon to be banished,

6 As Baker and Katz describe, 'BCG is the most controversial, as well as the oldest, vaccine in current use' because estimates of efficacy have ranged so widely, especially for protection against pulmonary disease – although it does appear to provide protection against tuberculous meningitis and disseminated disease in infancy (2004, p. 349).

so much so that the World Health Organization (WHO) passed a resolution in 1988 to eradicate polio by 2000 (Hajj Hussein et al. 2015). This three-decades-long drive has left only two countries where polio is still endemic[7] – Pakistan and Afghanistan – but the final push for eradication is proving difficult, especially following a 2022 resurgence of wild poliovirus (Rana et al. 2022).

By the 1970s, attention in the United States and Europe had turned to the so-called lifestyle diseases of civilisation, or more technically 'noncommunicable diseases', such as heart disease and cancer. However, the emergence of the human immunodeficiency virus and acquired immunodeficiency syndrome (HIV/AIDs) in the 1980s was a jolt to reality (Greene, Condrau, and Watkins 2016). As health researcher Peter Washer puts it: 'The meanings attributed to AIDS marked a break with history in that it ended the widespread twentieth-century optimism that modern biomedicine could offer freedom from fear of infectious disease' (2010, p. xii). Washer describes how the new field of emerging (and re-emerging) infectious diseases (EIDs) began to take shape from the late 1980s onwards, through conferences, publications, a dedicated journal, and the involvement of journalists (ibid.). Popular books captured the public imagination (e.g. Laurie Garrett's *The Coming Plague* and Richard Preston's *The Hot Zone*), influencing policymakers, funders, and citizens so that EIDs found a place high on scientific and political agendas. Vaccines also reached prominence in global health through the Expanded Programme on Immunization (EPI), which had been established in 1974 to develop child immunisation programmes throughout the world (Keja et al. 1988). As sociologist Stuart Blume (2017) notes, by the 1970s, public and social reactions to vaccination, including multiple vaccine controversies, were arising in response to political and technological developments related to vaccines across both lower- and higher-income countries. He argues that vaccination has been controversial as a technology, in public policy, and in the questioning by public groups since the very beginning. These developments make the history of vaccines not just one of responses to emerging and re-emerging

7 'Endemic' is when a disease is found regularly in a sustained community transmission for particular people or in specific geographic areas.

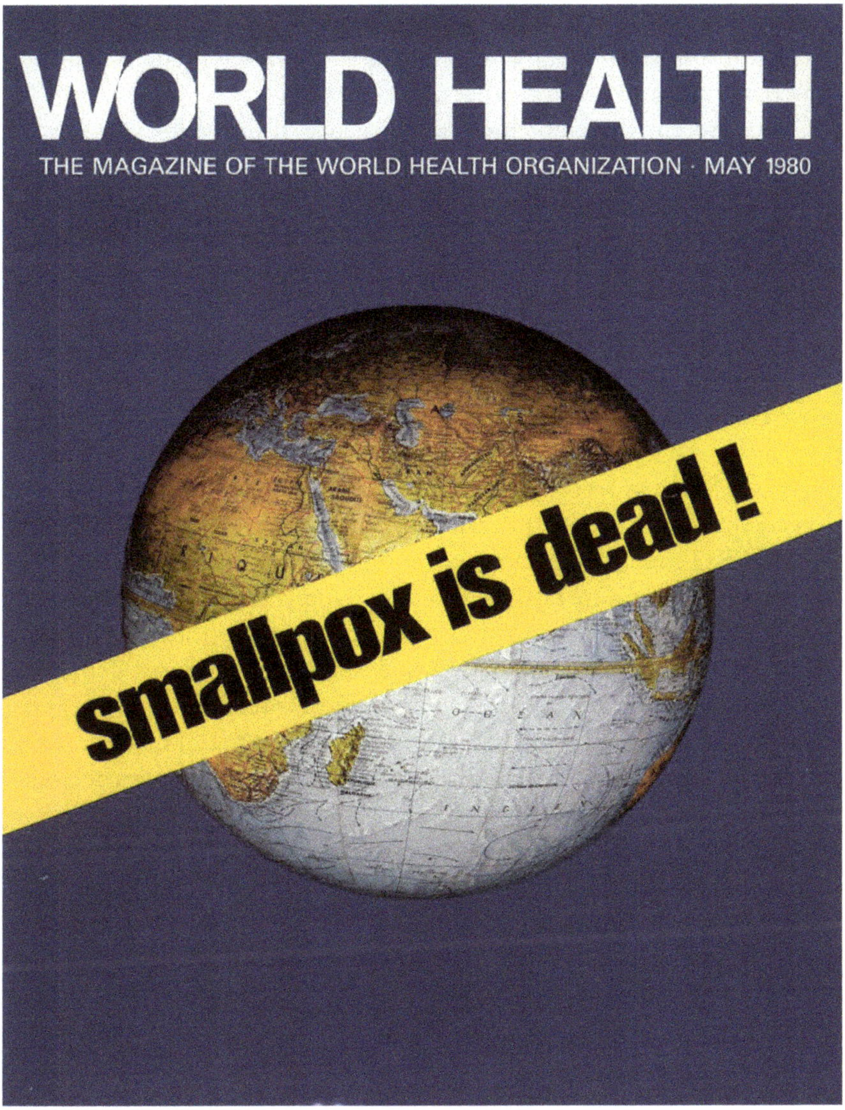

Image 1.3 Cover of *World Health* magazine (1980).

WHO (1980). Smallpox is dead! [full issue]. World Health, (May), 3–39. World Health Organization. <https://www.who.int/news-room/spotlight/history-of-vaccination/history-of-smallpox-vaccination>

diseases, which have been important in determining the vaccine landscape, but also one of new societal discussions of which diseases ought to be prevented, in what ways, and at what cost.

More recently, even before the emergence of COVID-19, a growing fear of global epidemics or pandemics was raised by public health commentators. These centred on EIDs, including HIV/AIDS, swine flu, and severe acute respiratory syndrome (SARS), as well as the potential re-emergence of old threats. At each juncture, the development of vaccines has been viewed with hope and as the best route out of an infectious disease crisis. Furthermore, the development of new technologies in molecular biology and advanced chemistry techniques which began in the 1980s led to improved vaccines in the 2000s (against hepatitis B, influenza, pneumonia, meningitis, and septicaemia) culminating in the recent COVID-19 vaccines being developed in record time (Almond et al. 2020).

As the COVID-19 pandemic has shown, vaccines can be objects of high public interest, and it was not long after the pandemic began that hopes for a vaccine were raised. Even then-United States president Donald Trump, who could be described as a former vaccine sceptic in his previous statements insinuating a link between vaccination and autism, demanded a coronavirus vaccine, saying: 'Do me a favor, speed it up, speed it up' (Thorp 2020). On the one hand, those who are critical or opposed to vaccination face a real-life reminder of a time before vaccines controlled many diseases, and this can prompt acceptance. On the other hand, there are also voices, which included celebrities and high-profile personalities, speaking about their unwillingness to be vaccinated, even before a vaccine is available. Such opinions face a greater chance of pushback from others when the stakes are higher in outbreaks. For example, the British rapper MIA attracted controversy for her tweet: 'If I have to choose the vaccine or chip I'm gonna choose death. YALA.'[8] MIA experienced a significant backlash from many followers who disagreed with her views (Image 1.4).

8 Posted on MIA's Twitter status: <https://twitter.com/MIAuniverse/status/1242788551563128833?s=20>. Note that YALA is an acronym for 'you always live again', a reference to the Hindu belief in reincarnation and a parody of the acronym YOLO ('you only live once').

The heightened reality of a very present disease threat may be the reason for a stronger countering by those who are in support of vaccination. A vaccine opposition constituency could have been seen as politically attractive

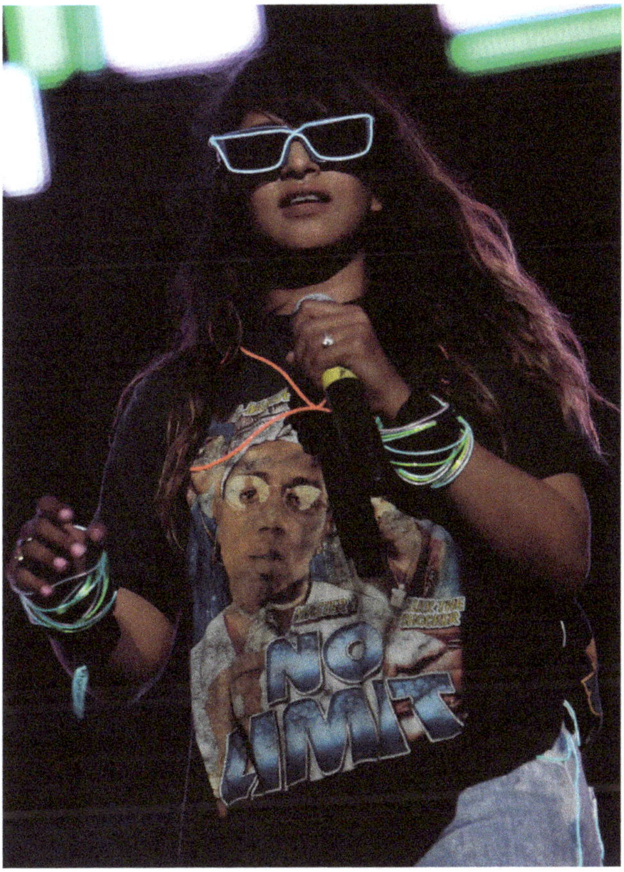

Image 1.4 British rapper MIA.
Steve C. Mitchell/EPA.

in pre-coronavirus times, but during the pandemic, vocal vaccine critics looking for votes found it difficult, as a Vermont governor candidate discovered when his stance against government-mandated vaccination was questioned by opponents (Thompson, Otterbein, and Ollstein 2020).

Vaccine-preventable diseases

The development of vaccines as biomedical intervention is shaped and imagined through society and public policy, marked by panic, misinformation, and a crisis of expertise, which came to the forefront with the COVID-19 pandemic. The eventual rollout of COVID-19 vaccines, as with many other vaccination campaigns, has been unequal both in supply and adoption. Still, it is not only during pandemics that this character of vaccines as biomedical interventions embedded in society becomes evident. Before the COVID-19 pandemic, regions across the world were already experiencing resurgences of vaccine-preventable diseases (VPDs), partly due to a fall in vaccine coverage.

VPDs form a disease grouping of common and serious infectious diseases for which an effective preventative vaccine exists, with the emphasis being on targeting children for immunisation through national routine immunisation schedules (WHO 2015). The situation that is commonly presented is one where the supply of vaccines by governments and the philanthropic sector means diseases can be controlled or even eradicated. Such optimism in vaccination, along with other medical inventions, follows the view that infectious diseases are deemed to be wholly conquerable. However, it is important to keep in mind that while these diseases have the potential to be controlled or even eradicated through technological innovation, what is feasible from the vaccine itself as well as implementation and social acceptance pose challenges. Also, the label VPDs is something of a misnomer as not all of the vaccines for VPDs identified by the WHO and in other standard lists are capable of preventing disease well. Box 1.1 shows the WHO's current list of VPDs.

Some vaccines may be safer and more effective than others. Vaccines have not always been developed through testing on the relevant populations where the diseases are most prevalent. There is evidence that in certain geographic areas children have a less robust response to the oral polio vaccine, the first Hib (*Haemophilus influenzae* type b) conjugate vaccine, and some rotavirus vaccines (Poland, Jacobson, and Ovsyannikova 2009). They may protect against one strain of a disease but not others. Moreover, all target groups in a population may not be protected. Indeed, neglect of some VPDs over others has meant that vaccines have not improved for many diseases because of a lack of market and donor interests. For example,

Box 1.1 World Health Organization (WHO) list of vaccine-preventable diseases

1. Cholera
2. Dengue fever
3. Diphtheria
4. *Haemophilus influenzae* type b
5. Hepatitis A
6. Hepatitis B
7. Hepatitis E
8. Human papilloma-virus
9. Influenza
10. Japanese encephalitis
11. Malaria
12. Measles
13. Meningococcal disease
14. Mumps
15. Pertussis
16. Pneumococcal disease
17. Poliomyelitis
18. Rabies
19. Rotavirus gastroenteritis
20. Rubella
21. Tetanus
22. Tick-borne encephalitis
23. Tuberculosis
24. Typhoid fever
25. Varicella and herpes zoster (shingles)
26. Yellow fever

Source: WHO (2017).

typhoid vaccines until very recently were primarily intended to protect the military and foreign travellers, and limit acute outbreaks (Kirchhelle and Vanderslott 2019a). The unevenness of what is vaccine-preventable or not is split along the lines of affluence, as well as the availability of preventative interventions, treatments, monitoring, and health systems. Such issues about the supply and access of vaccines worldwide are not given the focus they deserve, along with other factors that affect vaccination rates that are not addressed sufficiently, such as the provision of immunisation services by governments and access to available vaccines.

Misdirected attention is also problematic when the emphasis is on the people who oppose vaccination. The so-called 'anti-vaxxer', describing those that oppose, resist, or refuse vaccination, has become a figurehead to point to as the reason for falling vaccination rates. Anti-vaxxers can be a target for those looking for enemies in times of crisis, and this can fuel tensions and polarisation but they are not the unique explanation for low vaccination rates, and their influence is exaggerated in media portrayals, which rarely give a full account of a complex situation (Vanderslott 2018). The amplification of anti-vaccination views online and through the media, which has presented minority views as widespread, has led to false balance and increased polarisation (Ellerton 2014). However, when vaccination sharply drops, this is often connected with a particular controversy, event, or change of political environment, which tend not to originate from anti-vaxxer movements in particular. For example, measles is on the rise in Europe, and some places which until recently were considered by the WHO to have eliminated measles have since lost that status, as happened to England in 2018 (gov.uk 2022). Still, the highest number of cases over the past decade have been seen in Ukraine, a country that saw vaccination deprioritised after the fall of the Soviet Union and which has since undergone deep political turmoil and conflict, all contributing to poor vaccination services and a failing healthcare system (Kelland and Polityuk 2019).

Undue significance and a greater-than-warranted profile may be given to anti-vaxxers and an anti-vaccination rhetoric to present a bigger problem than actually exists and strawmen do not help in addressing the multiple problems that can cause low vaccination rates. However, this argument does not mean anti-vaxxers are harmless. People who are suspicious of vaccines, and especially if they openly tout their views, can be very harmful to public health. The worry of this is that even a small amount of persuasiveness coming from anti-vaccine narratives can have a magnified effect, given how rapidly a large part of the population may be exposed to such views (Curiel and Ramírez 2021). I will engage further with the specific use of the terms 'anti-vax' and 'pro-vax' and their effect in the next chapter.

The COVID-19 pandemic additionally demonstrated how people are being widely exposed to conspiratorial misinformation about vaccines, including stories about vaccines being 'a microchip or them being dangerous and harmful, causing death, or altering DNA' (Lee et al. 2022, p. 9). I follow the definition of 'misinformation' used by Herasimenka et al. (2022), which refers to any information that turns out to be inaccurate or false, and also includes 'disinformation' as a subset of misinformation, which is spread intentionally. Many have argued that online and social media misinformation has exacerbated concerns and trust in vaccines (Larson 2018). Such misinformation stories and messages are those that may contain useless, incorrect, or even purposefully harmful information and advice, which can hamper vaccine uptake. Misinformation anti-vaccine campaigns, particularly online and through the use of social media have taken the brunt of the blame for drops in vaccine uptake and become a worrying new trend (Burki 2020).

However, the politics of vaccine opposition is complex, subjective, and emotional, and does not only involve those in opposition to vaccination. Even one of the most famous cases, which concentrated in Britain but spread to other countries, on the infamous measles, mumps, and rubella (MMR) vaccine controversy, is far from a clear-cut case of anti-vaxxer views. The MMR vaccine had been introduced in the United Kingdom in 1988, but controversy arose from a now retracted 1998 *Lancet* article by Wakefield et al. purporting a link between the vaccine and autism (Murch et al. 2004). The article retraction by the journal happened 12 years after publication and following a General Medical Council Fitness to Practise Panel conclusion that 'several elements of the 1998 paper by Wakefield et al. are incorrect', particularly the claims about how children were consecutively referred and investigations being approved by the local ethics committee (Lancet 2010, p. 445).

As general practitioner Michael Fitzpatrick wrote in the *British Medical Journal* (BMJ), the media response across newspaper, radio, and television at first exacerbated popular fears by portraying the lead author Andrew Wakefield as a maverick and martyr to later present 'extensive and overwhelmingly supportive of the case for the safety of the MMR vaccine' (2008, p. 479). The tide began to turn in the early 2000s, exemplified by the *Guardian*'s 'Bad Science' columnist Ben Goldacre winning the 'best feature' prize at the British science writers awards for an article that criticised

Wakefield and his anti-MMR campaign (ibid.) (Image 1.5). However, it was the *Sunday Times*'s investigative journalist Brian Deer who in 2011 thoroughly exposed what he found to be 'bogus data' behind Wakefield's claims, revealing how Wakefield had knowingly manufactured the appearance of a causal link with autism to launch a worldwide scare over the MMR vaccine.

Nevertheless, the damage had already been done, with parental uncertainty and questioning of the safety of the MMR vaccine having led to a

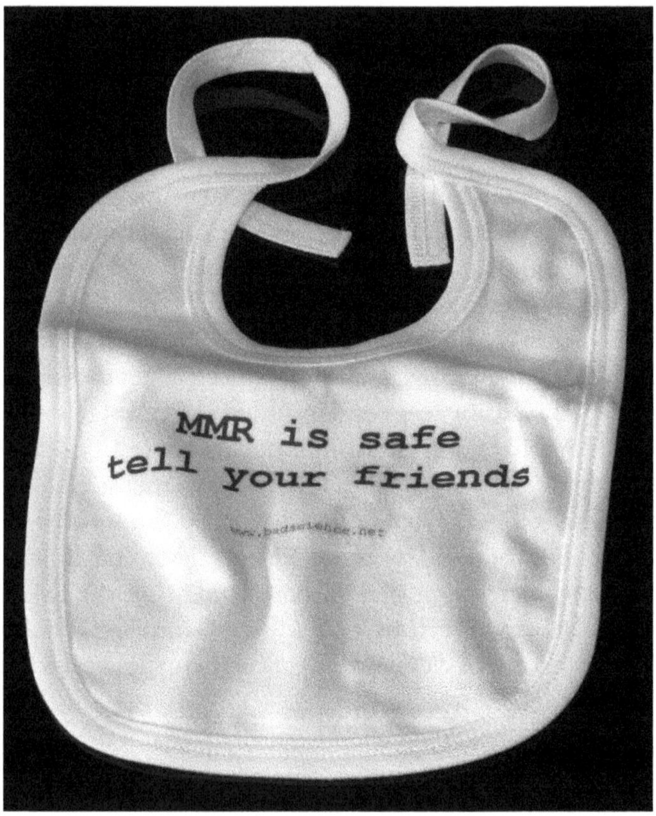

Image 1.5 Child's bib printed with 'MMR is safe, tell your friends'.

Science Museum Group. 2007. Science Museum Group Collection Online. Accessed 11 February 2023. <https://collection.sciencemuseumgroup.org.uk/objects/co8088846/childs-bib-printed-with-mmr-is-safe-tell-your-friends-bib>

dramatic fall in uptake. Outbreaks of measles were later reported in Dublin in 1999 and Swansea in 2013, leading to four deaths (McBrien et al. 2003; BBC News 2013b). This is an example of medical practitioners and researchers raising questions about vaccination and the public confusion that followed, compounded by media representation and mis-handling by public health authorities.[9] Still, media actors through journalists Goldacre and Deer can be credited with correcting misrepresentation. Indeed, historian Elena Conis (2015) has argued that concerns about a possible link between vaccines and autism were already brewing for years before the famous scandal, often coming from the autism community itself looking for explanations for a condition that lacks full explanation. The fear of autism being caused by vaccination continues even today, with public health authorities regularly needing to produce messaging about MMR vaccine safety (Image 1.6).

Vaccine support

Vaccines represent an opportunity for control through a 'magic bullet' – an idea stemming from the early 1900s proposal by German doctor and scientist Paul Ehrlich on the ability of drugs to target specific pathogens (Valent et al. 2016). The idea of a magic bullet has persisted as a cultural one of technological solutionism and was even made into a 1940 biological film about the life of Ehrlich (Tomes 2002) (Image 1.7).[10]

However, for mass vaccine campaigns to work magic bullets alone are not sufficient, and systems-building and societal support are also important.

9 Similar circumstances have been seen for other vaccines. For example, Japan suspended their recommendation for the Human papillomavirus infection (HPV) vaccine in 2013. It ignited public concerns about the safety of the vaccine in nearby countries such as the Philippines and in even more distant countries such as Kenya, where there exists a persistent fear about the government introducing fertility control through health interventions (Larson et al. 2014).

10 Released by Warner Bros., the film caused controversy because it covered the topic of syphilis, which was stigmatised as a sexually-transmitted disease, with Ehrlich

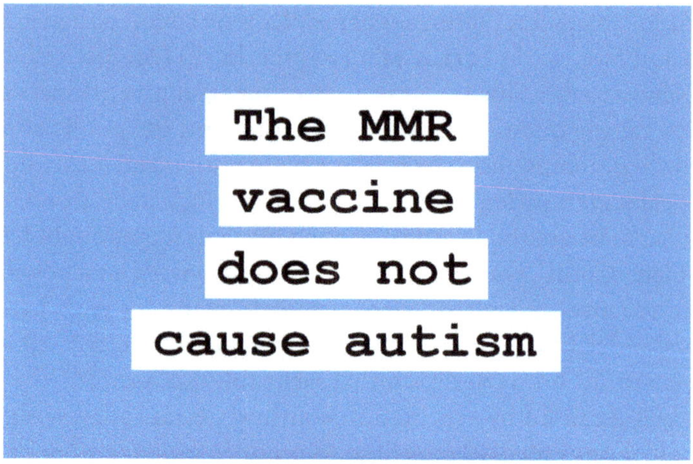

Image 1.6 MMR blog post by United Nations Children's Emergency Fund (UNICEF) Montenegro.

Emir Dresevic, UNICEF young reporter, The MMR vaccine does not cause autism, Fact checking, UNICEF Montenegro, blogpost. <https://www.unicef.org/montenegro/en/stories/mmr-vaccine-does-not-cause-autism>

Such a 'civil society' to advance the interests and will of citizens for vaccines is needed, and not only in high-income countries with advanced health infrastructure. Vaccines hold the hope for disease control and eradication; yet they can also provoke extreme societal reactions through deep-rooted concerns of harm and threats to liberty. This emotional discourse of hope and fear shows how vaccines are targets of various types of public attention as well as the need for safeguards and assurance from governments.

Global health scholars have made significant contributions to research on such public attention and vaccine governance (Verger et al. 2015;

depicted developing the effective treatment for the disease with Alfred Bertheim and Sahachiro Hata in the early 1910s. Salvarsan, also known as compound 606 and now more commonly as arsphenamine, is also used to treat relapsing fever and African trypanosomiasis. The film received critical acclaim and the screenplay was nominated for an Oscar.

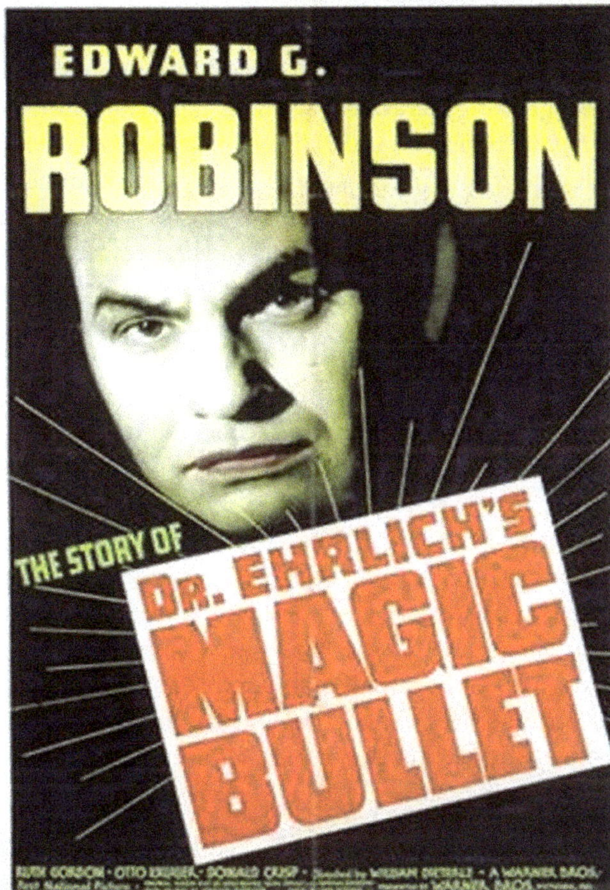

Image 1.7 US theatrical poster of *Dr. Ehrlich's Magic Bullet* (1940).

Fair use, via Wikimedia Commons.

Vignaud and Salvadori 2019; Carey et al. 2019; Larson et al. 2016a; Sridhar and Batniji 2008). Public policy research in particular has addressed why and how problematisation has evolved with new health threats and the potential of preventing diseases with vaccines (Shiffman 2009; Abeysinghe 2015). This literature considers both how private and social issues become collective public concerns to raise interest among policymakers, and the nature of conflicts related to science and technology in society, underlining the role of scientific reasoning and public input on topics of debate. Furthermore, a growing literature is also seeking to transition from public understandings of science to public engagement with science.[11] Still, what this scholarship does not directly address is how support for health issues is developed and promoted, and how this also draws on underlying conceptions about vaccines to identify the drivers and barriers for vaccine support concentrating on civil society advocacy and activism.

Civil society is an elusive concept that is difficult to define, mainly due to the heterogeneous actors involved. I use Anheier's working or operational definition because it emphasises collective organising that is rooted outside of the government or health professional sphere (Box 1.2). Turning the gaze away from opposition and towards support, vaccination appears as an important yet contested public health issue that has been subject to an underestimation of civil society activity (Vanderslott 2019). While much attention has been granted to those who oppose vaccination, support for vaccination is left out of the spotlight. Who are the so-called silent majority that contributes to the ongoing development, testing, and mass roll-out of vaccines? Concentrating on supporters, including pro-vaccine activists who campaign for vaccination, is an attempt to highlight vaccine support and provide further distinction about what this means from a civil society perspective.

Box 1.2 Definition of 'civil society'

Civil society is the sphere of institutions, organizations and individuals located between the family, the state and the market in which people associate voluntarily to advance common interests. (Anheier 2013)

11 For example, in the approach taken by Whatmore and Landström (2011) to modelling flood risk.

This book aims to shine a light on stories of advocacy and activism, through societal influence, media representation, and policy change, by public and professional vaccine proponents from parents, healthcare workers, to trial participants who provide their bodies to test new vaccines. In the following chapters, I present examples of support for vaccination through four examples to make diseases 'vaccine-preventable': (1) meningitis parent petitions; (2) pro-vaccine activist groups against measles and pertussis; (3) typhoid human challenge trials; (4) COVID-19 vaccine trials during a pandemic. These depictions of the civil society backing of vaccination are based on my own research about vaccine attitudes as a health sociologist, and on an analysis of different campaigns to explore pro-vaccine views and behaviours, including the aims and methods of engagement that are employed. My contention is that we can gain from reflection on such active civil society support, an aspect of vaccination that has been overshadowed by worries about anti-vaccine beliefs and behaviours. Therefore, I highlight less considered means of social organisation and document the views of vaccine supporters using mixed methods, and especially qualitative research, with principal methods employed being documentary analysis and semi-structured interviews. Public trust in science and health interventions faces ongoing challenges, especially when conspiracy theories and other online influences are so compelling. How civil society advocacy contributes to vaccine development, deployment, and acceptance deserves a more detailed exploration.

CHAPTER 2

Tracing Concern with 'Pro' and 'Anti' Positions

'Pro' and 'anti' positions for vaccination are labels often used without further distinction, which negates the complexity of the opinions and implies that there is an even split between two ideologically opposed camps (Ellerton 2014; Thomas, Tandoc, and Hinnant 2017). On the one hand, the 'pro-vaccine' or 'pro-vaxxer' categorisation is commonly used in mass media, policy, and academia, but it has not been problematised to the extent that the 'anti-vaccine' or 'anti-vaxxer' categorisation has. On the other hand, anti-vaxxers tend to be seen as personifying the problem of low vaccine uptake (Kata 2012; Venkatraman et al. 2015), amplified by anti-vaccine enclaves and echo chambers online (Kate, Chatman, and Martin 2016; Grant et al. 2015). However, some variation within is recognised. For example, social scientist Pru Hobson-West (2007) distinguishes between 'radicals', who reject vaccines outright, and 'reformists', who look to change vaccination policy. It is interesting that Hobson-West has observed with reformist parents the prevalence of personal experience where they believe their child to be vaccine-injured, and so while some are supportive of vaccination generally, they campaign for compensation, treatment, and better recognition of the dangers of vaccines (ibid.).

However, the meaning of 'anti-vax' (along with anti-vaccination, anti-vaccine, and anti-vaxxer) is a term used often without considering what is precisely meant. Very generally, it signifies opposition to vaccination and has negative connotations. I refer to anti-vaxxers as those who oppose, resist, or refuse vaccination, but opposition occupies a wide scope connected to a lack of trust or confidence. This position against vaccination is distinguished as being stronger and committed – as Burgess et al. (2021) describe, it is being 'wholly opposed'. The perception is of entrenched, unmovable views rooted in mistrust, for which there is little use in trying to persuade or convince otherwise. Refusal is more closely connected to a follow-up through behaviour, therefore, in not vaccinating. Again, this may not apply to all vaccines that are recommended. In contrast, the terms 'vaccine hesitancy' and 'vaccine-hesitant' concentrate on delay in acceptance and having questions and concerns, which can be addressed through better information, education, and engagement. Other researchers have identified a larger group of parents who can best be described as 'anxious' (Leach and Fairhead 2007) or 'hesitant', where they delay vaccination or pick and choose vaccine schedules, with skepticism as the driving force (Dubé et al. 2013b; Yaqub et al. 2014). However, most of the time, refusal is also included in this definition, such that vaccine hesitancy encompasses a broad spectrum of views (Moore et al. 2022). The delay in acceptance may also involve reluctance to accept standard recommendations, such as spacing out vaccination or seeking out individual rather than combined vaccines.

The meaning of pro-vax (along with pro-vaxxers, pro-vaccine, pro-vaccination) has seen little exploration in comparison with anti-vax, and it is the focus of the research presented in this book. Pro-vax is often defined more by behaviour than by attitude. Therefore, a common benchmark is whether someone has had all recommended vaccines or whether a parent specifically ensures that this is the case for a child. For example, in one study about the pro-vaccine groups that expressed hesitant attitudes, pro-vaccination was defined as 'participants who vaccinated their children with all vaccines according to the routine vaccination schedule' (Hijazi et al. 2022, p. 3). The associated pro-vax behaviours in cognitive and behavioural science, therefore, are those of compliance determined by passive acceptance rather than active demand built on trust (Faasse, Chatman, and Martin 2016). Going beyond this, it is also people self-reporting as being pro-vaccine as part of their identity and as a particular viewpoint that they agree with. Here supporting vaccination means to agree with the ideas and aims of vaccination and to want these to succeed and is thus often rooted in campaigning, advocacy, and activism. Still, most of those associated with vaccine support are groups typically thought to have an institutional agenda, encompassing healthcare workers, scientists, and government or public officials. This is not exclusively the case, however, as there are members of these groups who do not see themselves as vaccine supporters, just as there are vaccine supporters in groups extending far beyond these typical ones.

Important actors are also found within the public mass media and in social media groups, with campaigners, activists, advocates, professionals from other sectors, high-profile celebrities, politicians, and community or religious leaders all playing vital roles. However, such identities are not fixed and unmoveable. As Wang et al. found, parents can hold pro-vaccine views for example and still partake in what is seen to be vaccine-hesitant behaviour in delaying or spacing out vaccines, as well as having 'sympathy for and tolerance of vaccine hesitancy in other parents' (2015, p. 6703). This chapter further explores the core meanings associated with the anti-vax and pro-vax actors and groups, spanning the key related concepts from scepticism and hesitancy to trust and confidence.[1]

Scepticism and confidence

Next, I trace discussions about anti-vaccine positions through the terms 'scepticism' and 'hesitancy' in more depth, before moving on to pro-vaccine positions through the terms 'confidence' and 'support'. These are contested terms; as psychologist Matthew Browne points out, 'vaccine hesitancy or vaccine scepticism have suffered from an unfortunate lack of consistency in their use' (2018, p. 2540). By widening the scope to include these terms, I aim to gain a better insight into the views and ideas that these positions are most commonly associated with.

Scepticism is a philosophical position that questions the possibility of knowledge (Beebee 2018) and, some argue, as a concept is an integral part of science itself, both as a driving force and as a mechanism for improving the overall quality of science (Schmid and Betsch 2019). The scientific process can be viewed as an inherently sceptical one, as any question must be answered through experiment and evidence, while doubt is raised until an answer is provided. Scepticism is also one of the four 'Mertonian norms'

1 Drawing on Vanderslott (2017).

proposed by sociologist Robert Merton (1942) as core aspects of the ethos of modern science, the other three being communism (associated with communalism rather than Marxist communism), universalism, and disinterestedness. Organised scepticism is an ethos of science, as argued by Merton, and before scientific claims are accepted, they should be exposed to critical scrutiny in their methodology and through institutional codes of conduct.

What is special about the term is that people with diametrically opposed viewpoints can both be sceptics, as it is merely an approach – a questioning attitude or a tendency to doubt claims based on belief or dogma. However, where scepticism can be problematic to the scientific enterprise is when science itself is equated with belief or dogma, rather than being recognised and established knowledge, grounded in scientific consensus. For example, sceptics can be driven by both scientific and pseudoscientific beliefs and practices. Pseudoscience employs only the claim or appearance of use of the scientific method – of conjecture, prediction, and experiment/empirical observation based on hypothesis – while not actually following it (Finn, Bothe, and Bramlett 2005). In Chapter 3, I take a detailed look at sceptics against pseudoscience who counter anti-vaccine views. As Schmid and Betsch (2019) argue, the use of scepticism is typically different for scientists, who employ the idea of 'functional scepticism', which involves a readiness to update their prior beliefs depending on research findings. Science deniers, they argue, use an 'unfunctional scepticism' and only accept evidence that confirms prior beliefs that contradict the scientific consensus (ibid.). Schmid and Betsch describe how science deniers can question 'scientific milestones' to spread misinformation, and they advise providing the facts about the topic or uncovering the rhetorical techniques of science deniers in response (p. 931).

Another view commonly associated with science denialism is vaccine denialism, seen to be the most extreme form of anti-vaccine views. A number of scholars have argued that vaccine opposition can be thought of as containing features of science denialism, through the way in which claims are made in discounting evidence, creating villains, and shifting blame to another (Hausman 2019). Psychologist Matthew Browne (2018) identifies multiple social factors that drive scepticism towards vaccines, including how the success of vaccination has made the benefits less obviously apparent and how social media provides new scope for the spread of alternative claims on purported risks. There are also underlying psychological motivations to the determinants of negative vaccine attitudes. Vaccine scepticism (and rejection) has been connected to adherence to complementary and alternative medicine (CAM), which is popular because it is 'intuitively satisfying, and through appealing connotations with purity, naturalness and positivity' (p. 2540). Browne also argues that vaccine scepticism can be rooted in a 'spiritual epistemology' and 'openness to experience', a trait it shares with other forms of science rejection, such as climate change denial. Hornsey and colleagues identified two different vaccine-sceptical groups within a Spanish population sample; here, most vaccine-sceptical were 'highly educated and expressed strong liberal tendencies', sceptical about other controversial topics (e.g. genetically modified crops and nuclear energy), and most likely to receive science news from the internet (2021, p. 992). The second most vaccine-sceptical group was 'young, poorly educated, and politically extreme (both left and right)' (ibid.).

Scepticism also shows that attitudes do not always translate into actions. Just because a person has concerns over vaccination or says they do not want to vaccinate does not mean they follow up with their behaviour –known in psychology as the 'attitude-behaviour gap' or 'belief-behaviour gap'. In surveys measuring vaccine scepticism, high scepticism is rarely matched by low vaccination rates, with explanation for this mismatch varying from social pressure to repercussions of not vaccinating, such as not being able to enrol a child in school (Wellcome Global Monitor 2018). I will discuss further such a mismatch on a country level next.

Country confidence

In 2016, Europe was found to be the least confident region globally with respect to vaccine safety, and France was identified as the most sceptical country in the world, according to the Vaccine Confidence Project survey (Larson et al. 2016b). However, following a 2022 survey, this situation was found to have improved – especially for measles, mumps, and rubella (MMR) and seasonal influenza vaccines – although confidence had dropped in Eastern and Central European countries (Figueiredo et al. 2022). Generally, despite scepticism, Europe still tends to have high vaccination rates, along with North America, Central America, and Asia. This success is due to easy access to vaccines.

Outside of these regions, Saudi Arabia is a notable example of a country that reached full coverage in 1990 through an expanded programme of immunisation alongside better education and increased wealth (Al-Shehri and Al-Shammari 1991). At the other end of the scale, the Indian subcontinent, sub-Saharan Africa, and South-East Asia have low vaccination rates largely due to poverty and limited access to immunisation services and health education. Countries with high vaccine confidence, therefore, may be constrained by poor immunisation services, which prevent higher coverage. If vaccination is not offered at a sufficiently high availability and standard, there is arguably less capacity for opposition. Still, there are countries where, besides technical and organisational constraints, political and social resistance has become a greater problem, such as in Afghanistan, Pakistan, Nigeria, and Syria. Jonathan Kennedy and Domna Michailidou (2015), two researchers in global health and development, have argued that resistance to vaccination in such countries is better explained by political conflicts. Vaccination is, therefore, linked to concerns over interference, control, and dominance by unwanted forces, whether internal or foreign.

Given Europe's mostly high vaccination rates, it could be expected that there is a corresponding belief among populations that vaccines are safe and important. But as noted, Europe has been a sceptical region and even small drops in coverage can have dramatic effects. European countries have experienced cases of disease not seen in decades, such as the continued spread of measles, and in 2015, the first case of diphtheria in Spain in 28 years (Jané et al. 2018). The fall of communism either saw the collapse of immunisation services altogether, such as in Georgia in the early 1990s, or vaccination becoming a lower priority, such as in Romania and Ukraine (Doshi et al. 2009). Low uptake and low confidence appear to match closely in Ukraine, and the country saw outbreaks of polio in 2015 and again in 2021, in part attributable to disruption caused by conflict

(Hill et al. 2022). Issues of disparity between resources and influence can also be missed at a local level. Low-income areas, where it is more difficult to get advice on child health and immunisation, explain some lower rates or unvaccinated pockets. This is especially true for minority groups such as Romani people in Romania.

Apart from lower uptake, scepticism is also a problem for governments if it materialises into public resistance to vaccine policy. Such public resistance has a long history that stretches back to the origins of vaccination. For example, in the nineteenth and twentieth centuries, the National Anti-Vaccination League, formed from a merger of smaller organisations in 1896 (Grignolio 2018), and was active in Britain. It used pamphlets to raise concerns that vaccines contaminated children through transferring the pus of strangers and the blood of animals, thought to render them vulnerable to disease (ibid.). Resistance was especially acute in response to the English government's compulsory smallpox vaccination programme through the Vaccination Act of 1853 (Porter and Porter 1988). The act made it compulsory for infants under three months to be vaccinated, enforced through local registrars who gave out vaccination certificates to parents of newborns, which had to be signed by a doctor (Image 2.1). Parents who did not comply could be fined or imprisoned (Clark 2004). Historian Nadja Durbach (2004) documents how in the late nineteenth and early twentieth centuries, an anti-vaccination movement emerged in England in response to the government-mandated smallpox vaccine, which at the time was painful and potentially dangerous. The unpopularity of the act, which was compounded by the Poor Law authorities being the agency charged with the responsibility of administering vaccination, led to its effective abolishment in 1907 (Williams 1994).

As philosopher Vittorio Bufacchi (2022) points out, early 'compulsory' vaccination should not be confused with 'mandatory' vaccination, even though the terms are often used synonymously and both imply restrictions that derive from a rule or order. Compulsory justifies the use of force, while mandatory merely adds a cost to certain decisions to deter people away from making them (ibid.). For example, the United States has mandatory vaccination legislation requiring specific vaccines for school attendance with exemptions to opt out for what are prescribed as valid medical,

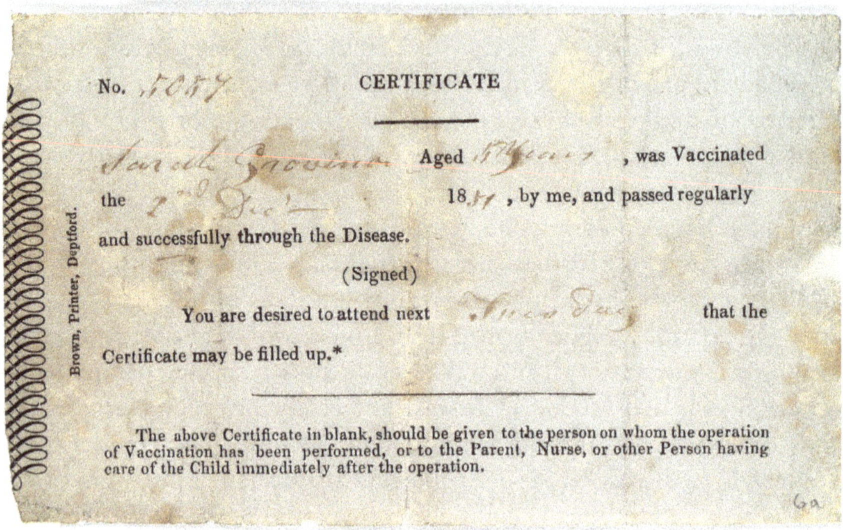

No. 5057 CERTIFICATE

Sarah Grovner Aged 5 Years , was Vaccinated the 2nd Dec 1817 , by me, and passed regularly and successfully through the Disease.

(Signed)

You are desired to attend next Three Days that the Certificate may be filled up.*

The above Certificate in blank, should be given to the person on whom the operation of Vaccination has been performed, or to the Parent, Nurse, or other Person having care of the Child immediately after the operation.

Brown, Printer, Deptford.

Image 2.1 Inoculation certificate for smallpox.

A certificate used by a patient, Sarah Grovner, aged 5, to establish that she has been inoculated to smallpox, on 2 December 1817. Wellcome Collection. Attribution 4.0 International (CC-BY 4.0).

philosophical, and religious reasons within the individual states. As of 2024, all 50 states offer medical exemptions, 47 states and Washington DC grant religious exemptions, and 14 states grant philosophical exemptions (for personal or moral beliefs) (National Conference of State Legislatures n.d.). Medical exemptions are given when a child has a medical condition that makes vaccination unsafe and prevents them from being vaccinated, while philosophical exemptions are given for 'conscientiously held beliefs of the parent or guardian', to take one example from Minnesota law (ibid.). Religious exemptions are given when vaccination is incompatible with religious beliefs, and some states ask for evidence of belonging to such a religious group. It is only Christian Scientists and certain faith healing groups (e.g. Church of the First Born advocates) that object to certain types of medical care and so maintain that vaccines are unnecessary (Kuru et al. 2022). The onus is placed on God rather than on vaccinations to prevent disease, coming from founding beliefs that viruses and bacteria are not the cause of disease (Swan 2020). Also, other religions have been associated with concerns about vaccine ingredients, including, for Muslims and Jews, the use of gelatin in vaccines; for Christians, the use of human fetal cell lines in vaccine development; and for other religious groups such as Buddhists, the treatment of animals (ibid.).

Today, countries have reconsidered mandatory vaccination once more in response to falling uptake, outbreaks of measles and other diseases, and, more recently, the COVID-19 pandemic. As described, the lower uptake has been associated with alternative views on lifestyle, education, medicine, and some religious beliefs. These subgroups may better explain outbreaks of diseases such as measles in Europe more than a widespread anti-vaccine movement. In recent years, France, Italy, and Germany strengthened and expanded their mandatory vaccination laws (Vanderslott and Marks 2021). For France, in 2017, 11 vaccines were made mandatory for children up to two years born from 1 January 2018 onwards. In Italy, six vaccines previously recommended (pertussis, *Haemophilus influenzae* type b, measles, mumps, rubella, and varicella) became mandatory in 2017 for children aged three to six, meaning 10 vaccines were now mandatory for minors up to age 16, with refusals facing fines and denied attendance of preschool. In Germany, measles vaccination became mandatory in 2020 for school and day-care attendance (it being illegal to homeschool children), as well as for other public spaces such as refugee shelters and clinics, with fines for non-compliance. Austria, Denmark, the Netherlands, and the United Kingdom also had measles outbreaks and discussed mandatory vaccination but did not implement it. Countries that imposed mandates during the COVID-19 pandemic included Indonesia, Micronesia, Turkmenistan, Austria, and Greece (Vanderslott 2021).

Defining and addressing hesitancy

'Vaccine hesitancy', a related term to scepticism, has gained popularity in recent years and can be traced back to parental acceptance issues for polio vaccines in the 1950s (Jacobson 2010). Uptake of polio vaccines was a key moment in public health, and Jacobson argues that hesitancy was differentiated from opposition that occurred previously because it was not politically motivated. Bedford et al. (2018) also find early use of the term to describe clinicians who were reluctant to prescribe vaccines in the 1990s. In more general usage, vaccine hesitancy was increasingly used by clinicians and medical researchers in the 2000s to refer to parents who were not outright refusing vaccines but rather delaying, being selective, or expressing uncertainty (Smith and Marshall 2010). However, vaccine hesitancy is used in quite wide-ranging ways, some including vaccine refusers and some not.

Attempts to measure vaccine hesitancy began when immunisation officers in the United States developed attitudinal measures of vaccine hesitancy to use in population surveys (Robinson and Priedeman Skiles 2008). The aim was to bring further nuance to the extremes of pro or anti vaccine characterisations (Ophir et al. 2022). By 2014, vaccine hesitancy was institutionalised by the World Health Organization (WHO) Strategic Advisory Group of Experts (SAGE) on Immunization with their published report, which provided a formal international definition: 'vaccine hesitancy refers to delay in acceptance or refusal of vaccines despite availability of vaccine services' (p. 7). To better understand barriers to vaccination coverage, instead of just labelling parents as being for or against, hesitancy depicts a scale from acceptance to opposition (Images 2.2 and 2.3). The importance of vaccine hesitancy at the WHO was further confirmed when in 2019, the organisation listed it as one of the most pressing global health challenges (WHO 2019b).

An expanded definition has also come from MacDonald et al. (2015a) who defined vaccine hesitancy as behaviour influenced by psychological factors, but also pointed out that it is a wide-ranging and heterogeneous phenomenon that varies by context, location, and source of information. As Bedford et al. (2018b) describe, in general usage the term broadly refers to suboptimal vaccine coverage, including those who are not being vaccinated for more practical reasons, right across to those who outwardly refuse. Furthermore, there is some imprecision about whether psychological state or behaviour is being referred to. As the authors succinctly put it, the problem is a lack of clarity in terminology: 'Only an accurate terminology can give us a clear idea of where the problem lies, allow us to assess

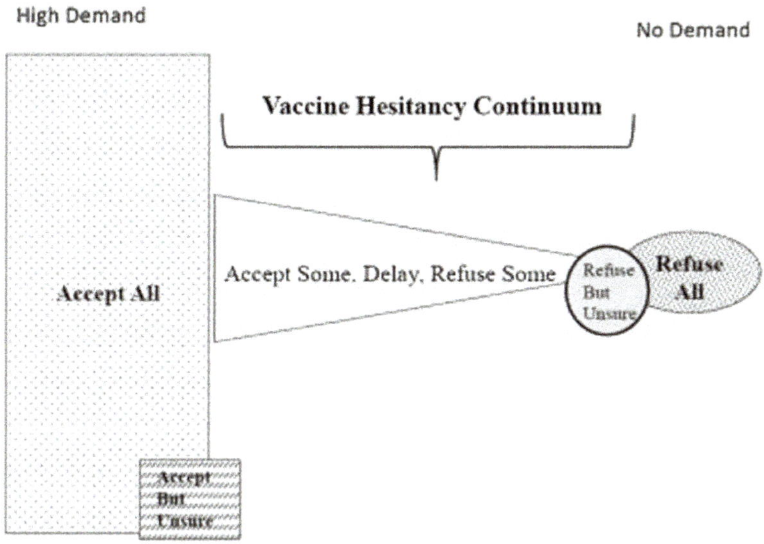

Image 2.2 Continuum of vaccine hesitancy from high to no demand.

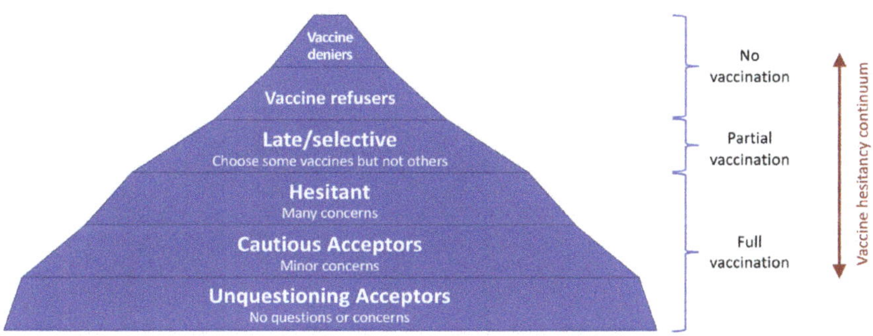

Image 2.3 Continuum of vaccine hesitancy from full vaccination to no vaccination.

its scale, and then focus our efforts accordingly' (p. 6557). Furthermore, as Kasstan (2021) points out, more often the problem is conceptualised as an attitudinal and behavioural one that emphasises people as problems, rather than looking towards other actors and the structural issues inherent in the production and governance of biomedical technologies.

Closely attached to the definition was the identification of a set of defining factors. Commonly used models of factors for vaccine hesitancy are the '3C' and '5C' models (Betsch et al. 2018) that relate, in particular, to relevant psychological concepts (Images 2.4 and 2.5). The 3C model was originally proposed in 2011 by the WHO EURO Vaccine Communications Working Group, where three categories – confidence, complacency, and convenience – were identified as factors affecting vaccine hesitancy (MacDonald et al. 2015b). Confidence is defined as trust in the effectiveness and safety of vaccines and the system that delivers them. Complacency exists where perceived risks of vaccine-preventable diseases are low and vaccination is not deemed a necessary

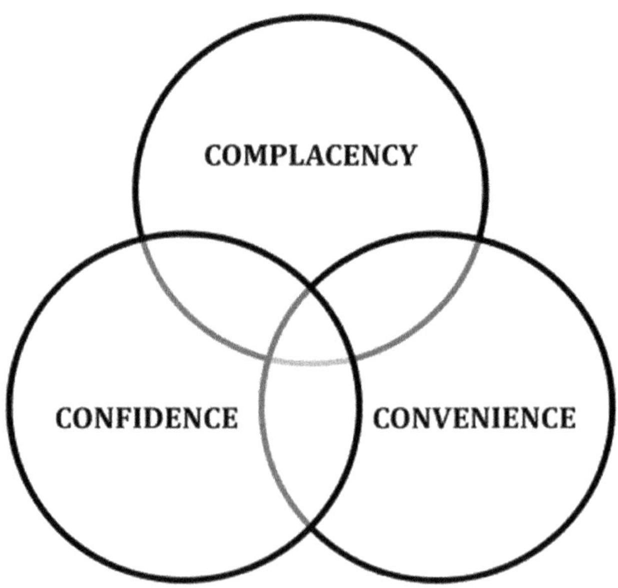

Image 2.4 The 3C model of vaccine hesitancy.

MacDonald et al. (2015a). Creative Commons CC-BY.

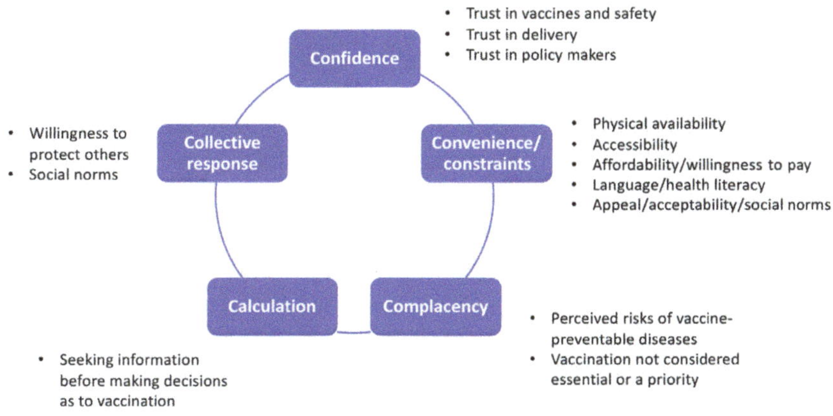

Image 2.5 The 5C model of vaccine hesitancy.

Turner et al. (2021). Creative Commons CC-BY.

preventive action. Convenience is when uptake is affected by physical availability, affordability and willingness to pay, geographical accessibility, ability to understand, and appeal of immunisation services.

Even though the term 'vaccine hesitancy' had strengths over previous concepts, it still proved problematic. The contested nature of vaccine hesitancy has persisted throughout its usage, but the term eventually took off and was adopted more widely by vaccine attitude researchers. Larson et al. (2014) made the argument that determinants of vaccine hesitancy had been focused on cognition-based features (knowledge, attitudes, and beliefs), drawing on commonly used classic health behaviour models.[2] They viewed the WHO definition of vaccine hesitancy as a positive step towards promoting a more appropriate and accurate terminology, as well as a method to understand why individuals and groups refuse vaccines, though also noting how the concept suffered from several drawbacks. Their contention was that vaccine hesitancy determinants did not adequately account for contextual influences to investigate the significance of social, economic, and/or environmental factors as determinants of health

2 The Health Belief Model and Theory of Planned Behaviour.

behaviour (sometimes called social determinates of health but spanning more widely). Behavioural and social science contributions have since concentrated on beliefs about vaccines (whether it conflicts with other beliefs) and views on benefits (perceived effectiveness and importance) or barriers (access and perceived risks). Furthermore, Peretti-Watel (2015) expanded their definition of vaccine hesitancy to a 'decision-making process', which alludes to it not being an endpoint but rather a state that persists until the point that a decision is made. Both of these contributions emphasise contextual influences. Models of vaccine determinants and factors, along with global surveys, have also been developed to include contextual influences, with an influential model by the WHO SAGE working group on vaccine hesitancy (Image 2.6).

The popularity in understanding lower vaccine uptake in terms of hesitancy has also followed through in the ways in which governments approach hesitant publics. One key intervention to address vaccine hesitancy has been through communication campaigns.[3] Public health communication involves both an explanation of official positions and efforts to increase community engagement, particularly targeting those who have displayed concerns or worries about vaccination. Another intervention is using carrot-and-stick policies to introduce rules to penalise, in addition to activities to encourage and persuade. Penalising policies include countrywide mandates for vaccination introduced by governments. In mandating such health interventions, often a balance between individual freedoms and collective goods is sought, and scholars have argued that a principle of 'least restrictive alternative' – implementing the lowest level of restriction necessary to achieve a certain public health goal – is the gold standard of public health ethics (Giubilini and Savulescu 2019). In addition, fairness in how freedom restrictions are distributed, that is, whose

3 There are a number of web resources that can be drawn on for vaccine communication from government websites for each country, as well as dedicated websites and within universities where more detailed but independent information, verified by experts, can be found: Vaccine Education Center at the Children's Hospital of Philadelphia (<https://www.chop.edu/centers-programs/vaccine-education-center>) and Vaccine Knowledge at the Oxford Vaccine Group based at the University of Oxford (<https://vk.ovg.ox.ac.uk/vk/>).

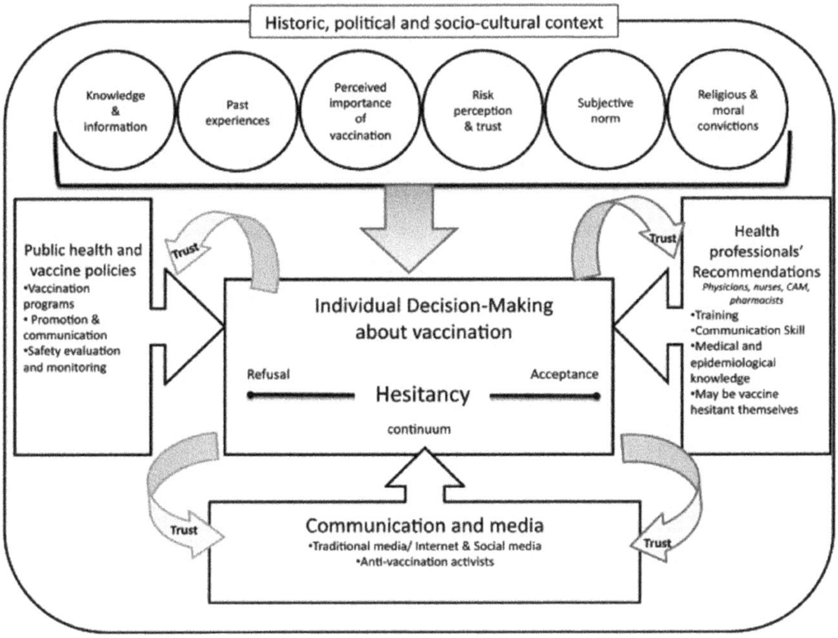

Image 2.6 Conceptual model of vaccine hesitancy.

Adapted from the Schema summary of discussions held during the workshop on the cultural and religious roots of vaccine hesitancy: Explanations and implications for Canadian healthcare. Dubé et al. (2013a).

freedom is restricted and why, is also an important consideration because the same freedom restrictions will affect different individuals and groups differently (Giubilini 2019).

Still, reaching such a balance is a challenge. The private sector in particular must contend with changing government guidelines as well as enacting their own business policies, which may also mirror government strategies in wanting to reward desirable behaviour through persuasion and penalisation. Given the complexity of vaccine hesitancy and the limited evidence available on how it can be addressed, identified strategies should be carefully tailored according to the target population, their reasons for hesitancy, and the specific context (Jarrett et al. 2015). While there is a lack of strong evidence to recommend any specific intervention to address vaccine hesitancy, multicomponent communication-focused interventions based on dialogue have been shown to be most effective (Dubé et al. 2015). As outlined by Ames et al. (2017), best practice emphasises clear and simple messages in a variety of formats adapted to the needs of each family, with clear answers to questions, made available at a wide range of health service and community settings. Time should be given to discuss and consider information and to ensure a supportive environment for decision-making that provides neutral information presented in a person's interests. One example of a specific approach is the C.A.S.E. (Corroborate, About me, Science, Explain/Advise) communication strategy, which can be used both online and offline (Jacobson and Rutten 2019). Strategies should be adjusted to respond to media stories, rumours, negative publicity and to answer questions or concerns.

Concentrating on anti-vaxxers

Even if the vaccine hesitant have received increasing policy interest, the media coverage and attention given to anti-vaxxers is disproportionately high compared to the actual impact they have. The parents who delay vaccination or pick and choose the vaccines they want make up a larger group, as one Canadian study found (Busby, Jacobs, and Muthukumaran 2017). Indeed, stories that have made the news include disagreements between parents that have resulted in high-profile court cases ruling in favour of the pro-vaccine parent (Volokh 2015) or penalties imposed by governments on parents not vaccinating their children, including preventing school entry in the United States or stopping welfare payments in Australia (Vanderslott and Marks 2021). The undue significance and greater profile given to anti-vaxxers makes them appear to be a bigger problem than they actually are. Presenting their views as more widespread leads to a false balance in the media and increases polarisation between those that support and oppose vaccination. False balance, according to philosopher Peter Ellerton (2014), gives a platform to views that do not have an equal weight of evidence supporting them, simply for the sake of appearing balanced. Relatedly, polarisation splits the debate into those who support an issue and those who oppose it (Mouw and Sobel 2015). There is not much room left for a variety of opinions in between, which makes it difficult for each side to find common ground or indeed any basis for discussion. Some in the media are attempting to move beyond this simplistic emotional narrative, but these sorts of accounts that tend to be longer and more investigative have become rarer.

There is already a long-standing discussion in vaccine attitudes research as to the extent of anti-vaccine views and whether it constitutes a social movement (Blume 2006; Hobson-West 2007; Ward 2016). The term social movement is problematic as it is difficult to demarcate from other types of organisational descriptors (Blume 2006), and a distinction must be made as to whether a movement is consistently, marginally, or occasionally vaccine-critical (Ward 2016). Social movements are commonly defined as intentional and sustained efforts to bring about or delay social change, usually outside of institutions endorsed by authority (Ritzer 2016). Additional understandings of social movements are of an organised and collective activity (Wilson 1973) and the sharing of a common culture (McCarthy and Zald 1977). Thus, anti-vaccine and hesitant views can be understood as a social movement that is a loosely organised but sustained campaign with long-term aims. However, vaccine views and behaviours are reflective of overlapping social, cultural, and political identities that cannot simply be distilled into an unproblematised binary distinction of either 'pro' or 'anti'.

Furthermore, anti-vaxxers do not offer a full answer for falling vaccination rates. Several reasons point to why people who have anti-vaccine beliefs and attitudes are not the sole cause of low vaccination. One is that anti-vaxxers are a small minority. The impression of most people is that this group is bigger than they actually are, when in fact the number of people explicitly not vaccinating tends to be very small (Kahan 2014). For example, in the United States, vaccine refusal is typically around 2 per cent (Seither et al. 2019). A similar rate is found in Europe, and these numbers have remained stable over time. One major fear is that anti-vaxxers may influence others, but vaccine acceptance is context dependant, for particular vaccines and at particular times and places as Dubé et al. (2021) argue. For example, a proportion of opposition against the human papillomavirus

(HPV) vaccine has been attached to moral concerns, as some parents feel that a vaccine against a virus that can be sexually transmitted is inappropriate for children (Bednarczyk 2015).[4]

Anti-vax portrayal

In allocating blame, if anti-vaxxers do not provide the full explanation for falls in vaccination rates, then why is the spotlight on them? While mainstream media is generally pro-vaccine, anti-vaxxers make for a good story, and this has been a feature from the early days of vaccination. Powerful imagery has been associated with anti-vaccine views. James Gillray's famous engraving 'The Cow-Pock-or-the Wonderful Effects of the New Inoculation!' (1802) demonstrated the fear of contamination with animal matter, even if done so as a satire (Image 2.7). In Gillray's caricature, people are sprouting cow heads after being innoculated in the Smallpox and Inoculation Hospital at St. Pancras. Another cartoon is a satire of the fear and distrust of vaccination by the French public, depicting a diseased woman who is turning into a mermaid, a physician who is riding a cow, and an apothecary wielding a syringe, to form a parade with the aim of scaring children (Image 2.8).

Satire of the fear of vaccination shows the perspective of vaccine opponents being ridiculed. Still, the overall effect is ambiguous as to whether their views are supported and also whether such views are amplified in this way. As Alex Green (2017) writing for the Wellcome Trust describes, 'It is hard to tell if these images are pro- or anti-vaccine, something which is often true of contemporary images.' There has also clearly been visual anti-vaccine propaganda, often distributed via pamphlets by anti-vaccine groups. A poisonous 'upas' tree (as a source of poison) was used as a metaphor for the effects of smallpox vaccination by anti-vaccinationists in the early 1900s (Image 2.9).

4 It is hard to find a powerful anti-vaccine group that has had a substantial impact, although one example is the 2017 outbreak of measles in Minnesota where a Somali community is reported to have been targeted by anti-vaxxers who saw potential to exploit this group using fears of the MMR vaccine and autism (Howard 2017).

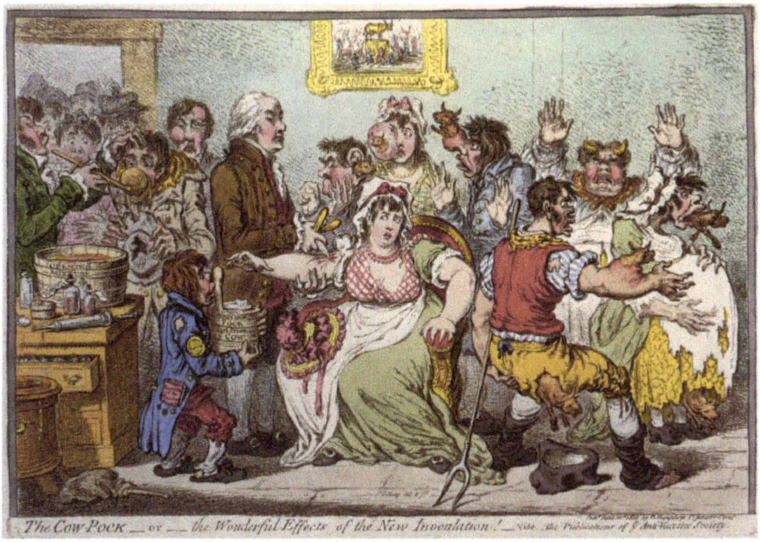

Image 2.7 The Cow-Pock-or-the Wonderful Effects of the New Inoculation!

Library of Congress, Prints & Photographs Division, LC-USZC4-3147. By James Gillray, 1802. Publications of ye Anti-Vaccine Society Print (colour engraving) published by H. Humphrey, St. James's Street. Public Domain Mark.

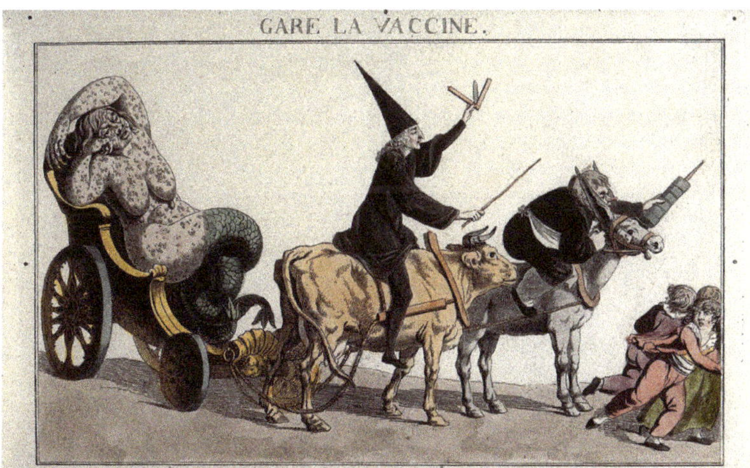

Image 2.8 Triomphe de la petitie verole.

Coloured etching c. 1801. Wellcome Collection. Public Domain Mark.

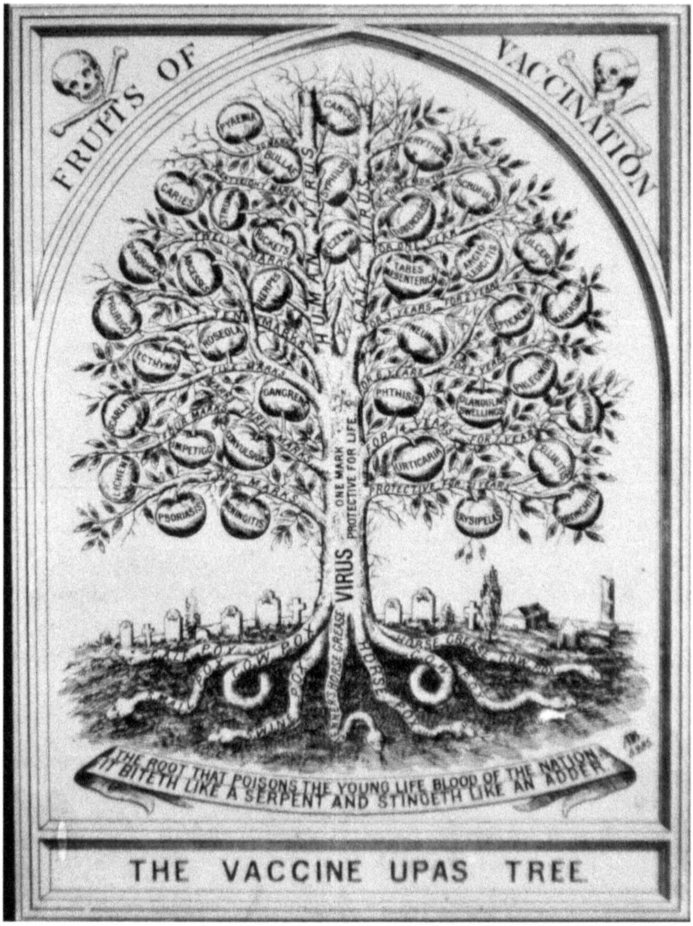

Image 2.9 The vaccine upas tree.

Early 1900s. The Historical Medical Library of the College of Physicians of Philadelphia. Public Domain Mark.

Instances of countering anti-vaccine views are also depicted in these cartoons, as shown in one etching, where there is a confrontation with each side holding giant lancets (a blade with a sharp point that was used as a needle) as weapons. Doctor Edward Jenner, a proponent of vaccination with two colleagues confront three anti-vaccination opponents who

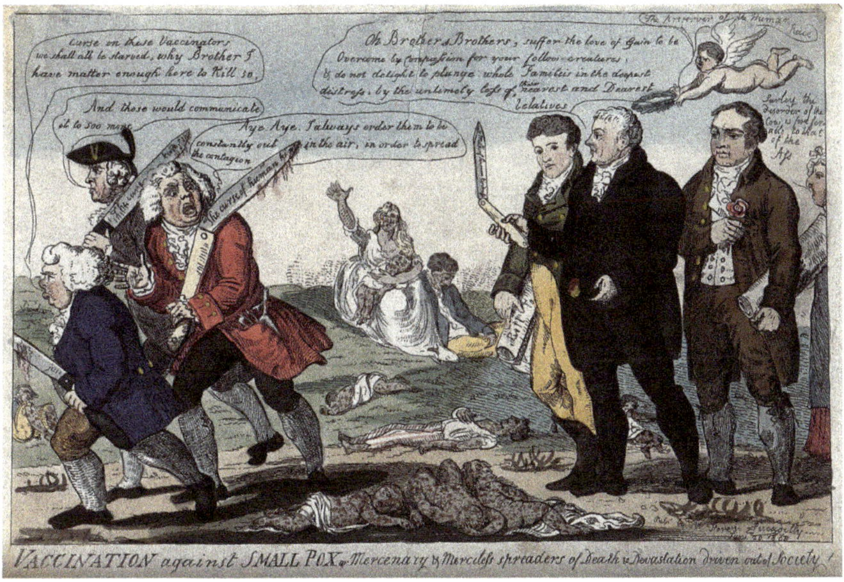
Curse on these Vaccinators we shall all be starved, why Brother I have matter enough here to Kill 50,
And those would communicate it to 500 more
Aye Aye. I always order them to be constantly out in the air, in order to spread the contagion
Oh Brothers Brothers, suffer the love of Gain to be Overcome by compassion for your fellow creatures, & do not delight to plunge whole Families in the deepest distress, by the untimely loss of their nearest and Dearest Relatives
The curse of human kind
VACCINATION against SMALL POX or Mercenary & Merciless spreaders of Death & Devastation driven out of Society!

Image 2.10 Vaccination against smallpox, or mercenary & merciless spreaders of death & devastation driven out of society!

Edward Jenner and two colleagues seeing off three anti-vaccination opponents; the dead smallpox victims are littered at their feet. 1808. Coloured etching by I. Cruikshank, 1808. Wellcome Collection. Public Domain Mark.

proclaim their anger at the vaccinators, 'Curse on these vaccinators' and speak of how they go about to spread disease: 'I always order them to be constantly out in the air in order to spread contagion.' The lancets of Jenner's opponents are labelled 'The curse of humankind', and Jenner asks for them to show compassion for others while being flanked by a cherub labelled 'The preserver of the human race'. The opponents are shown running away as explained by the title: 'Vaccination against smallpox, or mercenary & merciless spreaders of death & devastation driven out of society!' (Image 2.10). See Image 2.11 for a photo of the original Lancet owned by Jenner, which was used for vaccination at the time to make a cut in the skin.

The hidden issues and serious downside to attention on anti-vaxxers is that other issues remain unconsidered. With the concerns about vaccination

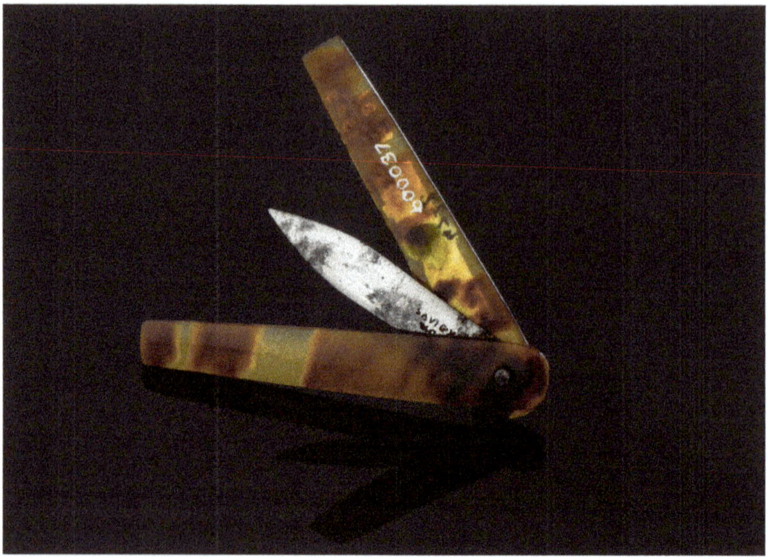

Image 2.11 Lancet belonging to Jenner, probably used for vaccination.

By Savigny and Co., 1701–1800, English. Science Museum Group Collection. A600037. Public Domain Mark.

opposition, what should not be neglected are routine immunisation programmes that protect people against vaccine-preventable diseases. The less attention-grabbing topics include poverty and exclusion, along with inadequate supply of and access to vaccine services, both on a global and a local level (Favin et al. 2012). However, the simple anti-vaxxer explanation is often preferred to a consideration of these more complex issues (Attwell, Hannah, and Leask 2022).

Furthermore, a narrative that concentrates on anti-vaxxers and constructs the public to blame for low vaccination rates acts to depoliticise rumours and increase mistrust during vaccination campaigns as well as deflecting wider challenges of a structural nature that determine vaccine uptake (Vanderslott et al. 2022). This treatment has persisted amongst vaccine decision makers, as Dutta et al. found in their recent study on their perceived barriers, which were outlined as located in communities for 'vaccine resistance, ignorance, lack of literacy, misinformation, confusion between vaccination and immunisation, logistics (remembering to get the vaccine), and relationships with the local health provider' (2021, p. 18).

Pro-vaccine actors and stories

The dominant narratives attached to anti-vaxxers are also true for pro-vaxxers. Pro-vaccine actors are typically thought to include governments and health authorities – healthcare professionals, in particular, are of high importance in communicating about vaccines because of the elevated levels of trust in them as an information source (Wellcome Global Monitor 2018). Not as widely reported on are activists, as Spier describes, and 'the successful prevention of disease in tens of millions of individuals is virtually ignored' (2001, S83). Still, pro-vaccine activists and their associated campaigns have reached some prominence. An example of a pro-vaccine activist in the public eye is Paul Offit (Image 2.12). He is an American paediatrician and co-inventor of a rotavirus vaccine. Offit is unusual in how engaged he is in the public sphere, authoring popular books on vaccination and appearing as an expert in the media and online (e.g. on Medscape, a medical news website). However, Offit reflects on how he is vilified. This treatment stands in contrast to other figures reviled for their pro-vaccine views. Jonas Salk, the inventor of the first polio vaccine, was celebrated as a national hero for his scientific achievement: 'When Jonas Salk invented the polio vaccine, he was a hero – and I'm a terrorist?' (Paul Offit quoted in McNeil 2009). At the height of his fame, Salk appeared on the cover of Time Magazine in 1954 (Image 2.13).

Offit, while outspoken, does not make overtly confrontational attacks on vaccine critics and is wary of taking any direct action aside from voicing his opinion. He mainly speaks out in support of vaccination through mainstream media and popular science books. In response, he is labelled as an anti-hero who threatens individual liberties through violence and fear – and is a regular target of online hate mail and death threats (Smallwood 2008). These experiences are indicative of how a scientist who developed a vaccine and espouses pro-vaccine views can be viewed as a negative force,

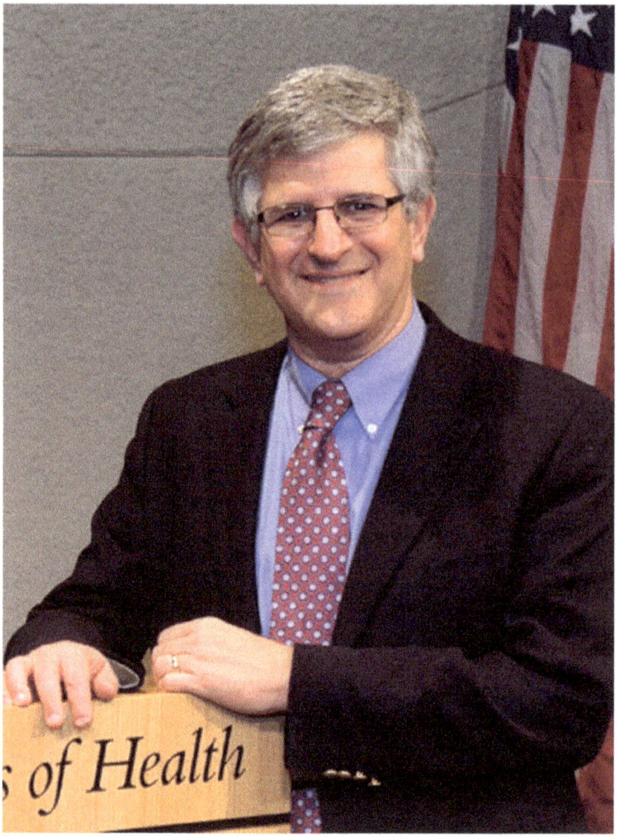

Image 2.12 American paediatrician Paul Offit.

Michael Spencer for the National Institutes of Health Record, Public domain, via Wikimedia Commons.

albeit by a small number of people. The comparison to Salk shows how, at various times, at various places, and for certain diseases, vaccination has been viewed, demanded, and supported very positively. When Salk's polio vaccine was successfully trialled in the 1950s, 'church bells tolled, horns honked, and sirens rang out as the nation rejoiced' (Jacobs 2015, p. 166). The mid-century was a 'golden decade of vaccines, when immunization became a "sacrament" that received only rare public questioning' (Johnston 2004, p. 244). The fear and devastation of polio saw parents lining up in the streets to have their children vaccinated in an outward display of support.

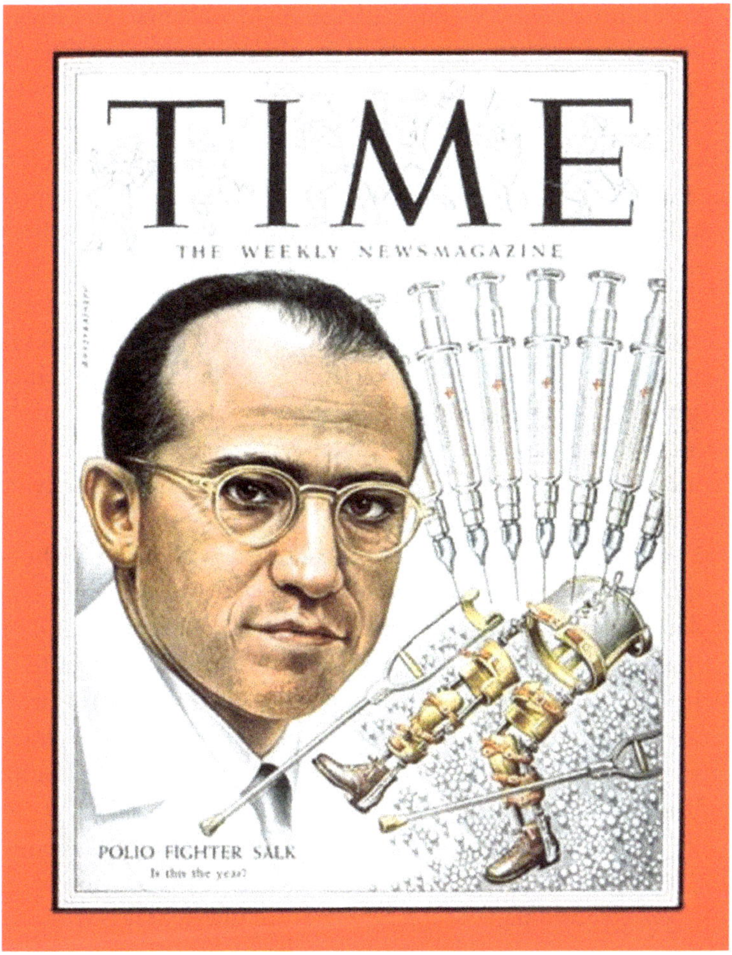

Image 2.13 Jonas Salk on the cover of *Time*.

TIME USA, LLC. March 29 1954. Cover: Boris Artzybasheff, Public domain, via Wikimedia Commons.

Pro-vaccine activism

The activities of pro-vaccine activists is an area of focus that has been overlooked in the past and deserves to be highlighted. Pro-vaccine activism is action that seeks to initiate change in vaccination by reinforcing the mainstream and (or) countering digression from it (Vanderslott 2019). I use the term to mean the citizen-led promotion of vaccination uptake that is proactive in seeking change. As Moskalenko and McCauley (2009) have argued, there is a scale of involvement in political mobilisation that makes the distinction between activeness and collectiveness in 'pro' activity important. By 'activeness', I refer to the level of direct action taken in support of vaccination and 'collectiveness' as to whether this is done in a group and for collective ideals. This is activism to promote vaccination organised at the citizen level, going beyond dominant social practices endorsed by authorities. While anti-vaccine activism has been widely documented and discussed, less has been said about the concerted response of pro-vaccine activists defending the majority view. These views and behaviours can take varying forms due to different aims and methods of engagement. Understanding public support for (as well as public opposition to) vaccination can help to give a better insight into views and behaviours, with wider implications for the study of counter-activism and the polarisation of civil society groups.

Pro-vaccine views did receive some scholarly attention in the 1990s. Anthropologist Mark Nichter (1995) originally distinguished between 'active demand' in an informed public recognising the need and benefit of vaccination, and 'passive acceptance' of the public yielding to health authority recommendations and societal pressure. Nichter proposed a contrast between the demand of informed publics on the one hand, and passive acceptance of publics whose acceptance of vaccination is a result of following authority on the other (ibid.). He used the concept of ignorance to explain acceptance and hesitancy, where the public's ignorance is posited to be a limitation on what they know or understand. The active and passive characterisation of Nichter is still relevant, as there are parents who actively demand vaccination just as there are others who actively resist it. Where less attention has been directed is what motivates or influences overt civil society demand and support for vaccination, either during times of opposition to vaccination or stable periods of vaccination uptake.

Pro-vaccine activism is difficult to assign a 'movement' character to as noted already in the difficulties of anti-vaccine activism in meeting the criteria of having a sharply defined issue that constitutes a new political identity (Blume 2006). However, much can be still drawn from the sociological literature of new social movements and, more specifically, of the health and social movements that have emerged since the 1960s in considering pro-vaccine activism. 'New' social movements focus on public and government relations, often taking the form of resisting control and challenging authority (Brown and Zavestoski 2004) and concern for 'identity, individuality and control of one's body', bringing those issues to wider acceptance by the public (McInerney 2000, p. 138). Pro-vaccine activism stands apart from the type of health social movement typically studied. These sorts of activists tend to emphasise group identification, collectiveness, and public control, without particular concern for popular acceptance (Maciuszek et al. 2021). Maciuszek et al. (2021) have made some pointed observations about the pro-vaccine groups behind such activism, in having a higher group identity than anti-vaccine groups, but with both groups having a positive attitude to science. This group dimension to vaccine decision making is novel, as research has concentrated mostly on individual differences. As Attwell and Smith argue, 'the decision to vaccinate or not is an inherently social one, and not a matter of individual rationality' (2017, p. 183).

The social organisation of pro-vaccine groups presents an additional aspect of support for vaccination, which has previously been relegated to government, policy officials, the medical establishment, and public health institutions to address and also counter anti-vaccine views (Dubé et al. 2013). While being a heterogeneous collective, pro-vaccine activists share a social 'health issue identity', as do those critical of vaccination, who have attracted the most focus in recent years. However, their activism stops short of what might be viewed as a fully-fledged social movement but rather reasserts an accepted view in line with government authority and control. What is valuable to take from this concept of health social movements, as Brown et al. (2004) have explored, is how identity is politicised and made collective. Identities are formed through the experience of the health issue in question, but also the political position this produces. Thus, the resulting identity is self-fashioned through the combination of biomedical and social worlds into one where the biomedical authority is still present, but the individual is not simply a passive receptor.

Online battles

Alongside healthcare professionals and activists, the internet is a central public resource for people to research health topics. For example, in 2018, a survey found that 75 per cent of Americans seek health information online (Weber Shandwick 2018), and there are over one billion health-related searches on Google every day (Murphy 2019). Vaccine-related material available online is of variable quality, however, and internet search engines can often direct web users to low-quality or anti-vaccine websites (Finnegan et al. 2018). The role of information provision by websites to mitigate the spread of misinformation becomes even more crucial during a pandemic. A large volume of inaccurate information about COVID-19 circulated since the beginning of the pandemic, for example, and has included misinformation about vaccinations against the infection.

The online sphere has therefore also become a discursive battleground between supporters and critics of vaccination. It is in this virtual space that pro and anti positions are increasingly being defined and redefined through social media and other online venues. This virtuality allows for networks to be created based on shared beliefs for narrow topics and gives organisers a resource-light means of sharing ideas and enabling discussion. Social media especially offers the means of putting forward opinions, helps to amplify views, and provides an organising space for action. For pro-vaccine supporters, this has helped turn a previously quiet and disparate constituency into an active online support for vaccination. The most influential content by both pro- and anti-vaccine proponents can be visual, for example, through memes (Harvey et al. 2019).[5]

Although anti-vaccine, anti-establishment groups initiate the spread of memes and form the core of many networks, as Lutkenhaus et al. (2019) found with mapping the Dutch vaccination debate on Twitter (now called X), there are also other clusters, such as evangelical Christian groups, as Rogers and Powe (2022) found, that spread politicised misinformation and act as bridges to disseminate memes at the regional or national level. This activity contrasts with other misinformation networks which are characterised by echo chambers (Törnberg 2018). Memes can also provide

5 Although studies about misinformation largely focus on text instead of images.

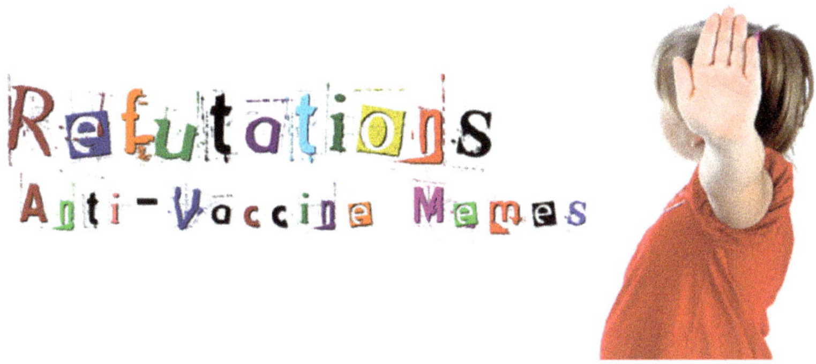

Image 2.14 Refutations to anti-vaccine memes.

Used with permission of owners. <https://www.facebook.com/RtAVM/>

a format for the pro-vaccine side to use comedy and satire as a tactic to demean and ridicule vaccine critics (e.g. a Facebook group called 'Refutations to Anti-Vaccine Memes' using humorous memes to counter vaccine critics (Imagee 2.14)). A similar approach has been taken on American online forums, such as the blog 'Respectful Insolence' by surgeon David Gorski, refuting pseudoscience claims. The attacks made are often identity-based in their character but do not directly attempt to disrupt the activities of vaccine critics.

The dangers of misinformation spread online presents more of a risk for certain groups, including healthcare workers because of their ability to influence others. As Verger et al. (2022) found, vaccine hesitancy in healthcare workers is rooted in a lack of knowledge about and mistrust of health authorities, the pharmaceutical industry, and experts. They recommend improved content about vaccination in training programs, better access to information in consultations, and instruments to measure vaccine hesitancy. However, advice has been lacking in how to address misinformation via online means. Vaccine attitude researchers also turned their attention to online social spaces relatively late. An in-depth view of the role of social media platforms for protest and social movement activity was generally reserved for other topic areas. Now a growing number of researchers, including Kata (2012) as one of the earlier examples, have explored online activities related to vaccine attitudes, particularly anti-vaccine misinformation. Moreover, organising online has greater influence on societal vaccination discussions and policy.

While vaccine hesitancy associated with misinformation was already a global health research priority identified by the WHO (2019b), it became a centrepiece issue in the COVID-19 response. The scope of online misinformation covered many aspects of the COVID-19 pandemic. Vaccine opposition discourse centred on mistrust of the speed and process of creating vaccines, and of the contents and micro-constituents of vaccine ingredients, including conspiracy theories about whether vaccines contained DNA-altering properties (for messenger ribonucleic acid (mRNA) vaccines such as Pfizer and Moderna) (Islam et al. 2021). Some also had beliefs about non-health-specific reasons to mistrust vaccines, such as that governments aimed to use COVID-19 to control citizens. These discourses often contained vaccine misinformation regarding vaccine side effects or vaccine harm, such as reduced fertility, chronic illnesses, birth defects or harm to unborn children, and risk to lives. These ideas circulated widely on social media and platforms have taken steps to address misinformation. Social media platforms were already aware of their role against fake news and company representatives met with government leaders early on in the COVID-19 pandemic. Although some platforms have more limited control and oversight, such as with private messaging such as WhatsApp, email, and text messages. Until recently, a function of 'frequent forwards' allowed content to be shared rapidly with multiple users; however, in 2019, WhatsApp decided it would limit the number of times a message can be forwarded to a maximum of five chats, including one group chat (Reuters 2019).

Online misinformation poses a challenge to public health and has prompted interventions, including using corrective information undertaken by the global health community, particularly during the pandemic. Activities to derail vaccination campaigns have occurred in the past, as in 2017, when a rumour that vaccination would make children impotent hampered the Indian government's vaccination campaign for a new measles and rubella vaccine in five states (Rao and Govindarajan 2017).[6] Health

6 Explored further in Chapter 3.

authorities and governments need to react promptly to information that is false or misleading to address this risk. For example, the European Centre for Disease Prevention and Control (ECDC) launched a campaign in June 2021 to provide posters to promote vaccination information from trusted sources (Image 2.15).

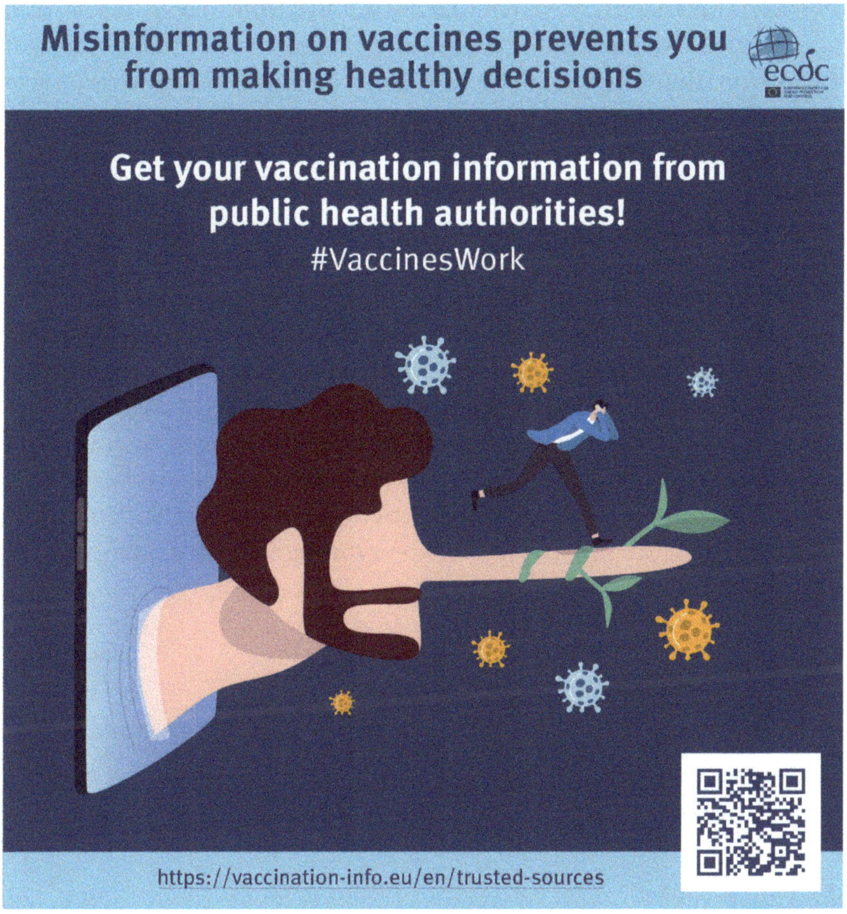
Misinformation on vaccines prevents you from making healthy decisions
ecdc
Get your vaccination information from public health authorities!
#VaccinesWork
https://vaccination-info.eu/en/trusted-sources

Image 2.15 The European Centre for Disease Prevention and Control (ECDC) vaccine misinformation poster.

ECDC (2021). <https://www.ecdc.europa.eu/en/publications-data/poster-countering-online-vaccine-misinformation-0>. Public Domain Mark.

A feature of communication during the pandemic has been the mixed, changeable, and unclear public health messaging or official advice regarding vaccination, along with officials acting as poor role models. As people have tried to make sense of COVID-19, the sharing of emerging research studies and impact of academic preprints on global discourse in the media and online led to considerable debate, and a worry about the reliance of policymakers on scientific research that has not had time to be peer reviewed or replicated (Majumder and Mandl 2020). Still, at its core the spread of misinformation often stems from scepticism about the motivations of those who have developed a new vaccine and may lead to questions about how safe and useful it is. Such a refocus on online information and misinformation as a key concern for both pro and anti positions has taken the labels and terms used in vaccination discussions towards wider structures of communication.

I have shown through this chapter the binary representations of 'pro' and 'anti' in vaccine discourses, the role of skepticism and confidence, and presented the problem of vaccine hesitancy. I discussed the attention that anti-vaccine views receive and introduced the idea of pro-vaccine activism and new challenges brought by the online sphere. However, it is important not to lose sight of the many other places that civil society has become active in with respect to vaccination, particularly in support of vaccination. This is what I address in the next chapter through detailed examples.

CHAPTER 3

Examples of Civil Society Support for Vaccination

Support for vaccination within civil society is gaining momentum, adding its voice to that of governments, health professionals, and other more traditional vaccine advocates. Four examples in this chapter describe pro-vaccine support over the past 20 years for the development of new or improved vaccines and policies to promote vaccine uptake for meningitis, measles and pertussis, typhoid fever, and COVID-19 across different contexts. I have chosen these four examples as most emblematic of different aspects of civil social action through public petitions (meningitis), activism (measles and pertussis), and trials (typhoid fever and COVID-19). The example of meningitis is a way to present more traditional means of advocacy through petitions and charities to garner vaccine support. Measles and pertussis present citizen activist examples. Typhoid fever shows the role of the trial participant alongside the advocacy of international organisations to bring public and policy attention to an overdue vaccine. COVID-19 situates trial participants as advocates within the representation and composition of trials during outbreaks. Such pro-vaccine public advocacy, support, and activism span predominantly childhood diseases (meningitis, measles, and pertussis) and those that have targeted older populations (typhoid fever and COVID-19). These demonstrations of pro-vaccine views have been under-researched in comparison with anti-vaccine views, and it is crucial to also take into account the institutional landscape of vaccination policy that involves a variety of actors from government, media, health authorities, and non-governmental organisations to wider publics.

Meningitis – a new vaccine for a feared disease

The development of a meningitis vaccine offers an example of how parent groups and disease charities, through social media and the use of online public petitions, worked together to galvanise support for the development and rollout of vaccines. I analyse this case by identifying the constituency that made up an ePetition (a petition administered online) in the United Kingdom in the early 2000s, the trigger that popularised it, and what success it had. Support for a vaccine has been in part because meningitis is a concern for parents – a bacterial or viral infection of the protective membranes around the brain and spinal cord, mainly affecting children and young people. The fact that it can be devastating if not treated quickly makes it especially alarming. The symptoms are well known, thanks to government and charity awareness programmes: a stiff neck, fever, aversion to bright lights, and (especially in later stages) a rash that does not fade when pressure is applied by rolling a glass over it.

Without prompt treatment, infection can lead to blood poisoning (septicaemia) and permanent damage to the brain or nerves or can develop into septic shock, resulting in death. A major cause of meningitis and septicaemia is invasive meningococcal disease (IMD), which has case fatality rates of up to 80 per cent in untreated cases and 4–20 per cent with appropriate treatment (Parikh et al. 2020). The high case fatality rate and potential for serious long-term complications has meant that meningitis is a feared disease, although incidence has declined in most parts of the world over the past 20 years, in part due to immunisation programmes (ibid). The seriousness and rapidity of meningitis infection make it a clear candidate for a vaccine, although this is complicated by the numerous serogroups associated, as IMD is caused by the *Neisseria meningitidis* bacteria, of which 12 types (or serogroups) have been identified.

In the United Kingdom, the four most common serogroups have historically been B, C, W, and Y, all of which can cause epidemics (McIntyre et al. 2012). The recently circulating meningococcal W (MenW) serogroup has been more aggressive, accounting for a third of deaths of those infected in 2017 and has caused an overall increase in cases of meningitis and septicaemia, with cases for example in England rising nearly tenfold from 22 cases in 2009–10 to 210 in 2015–16 (NHS n.d.). A vaccination for MenC disease was the first meningococcal vaccine introduced into the United Kingdom national schedule in 1999, following an increase in cases that occurred in the mid-1990s (Khatami and Pollard 2014). Work on these MenA and C vaccines had originally begun in the 1980s, with non-profit research organisation Sclavo Vaccines conducting the first human trials in 1991; however, the circulation of serotypes did have an effect on vaccine development, and the low prevalence of MenA in developed countries and increase in MenC infections meant that the focus was then switched to MenC (Snape and Pollard 2005).[1] As a result of MenC immunisation programmes spanning Europe, Canada, and Australia for over a decade, cases fell dramatically (Andrews and Pollard 2014). MenB then became the dominant strain affecting children in England, especially those under five years old, accounting for approximately 80 per cent of all laboratory-confirmed cases in England (PHE 2015). This was a worrying development as around a tenth of survivors of MenB disease will have major physical and/or neurological disabilities, and one-third will have less severe disabilities (ibid.).

The first vaccine for MenB took over 20 years to develop and licence – a relatively quick timespan for the development of a vaccine. For some diseases, it can take much longer, depending on the motivation to develop a vaccine and other circumstances. It not only requires the alignment of many different actors (including pharmaceutical companies, government departments and agencies, public groups and civil society, and international institutions and donors) but is a major scientific and technical endeavour, all under the pressure of potential markets or public health need. In addition, the social support for developing vaccines against meningitis has been important. Historian Baptiste Baylac-Paouly (2019), who works on the politics of vaccination in the twentieth century, argues that histories of vaccine development tend to concentrate on a 'history of progress' rather

1 Pharmaceutical companies Chiron and Wyeth then used a genetically detoxified diphtheria toxoid (CRM197) protein carrier, and Baxter used a tetanus toxoid carrier (Girard et al. 2006).

than highlighting these social factors. The development of MenA vaccines was a 'doable problem', according to Baylac-Paouly, because there was alignment between experiment, laboratory, and the social world as three levels of organisation. In the social world, a combination of collaborations, discussions, and trials are required, with a network of supporting relationships. A similar story can be traced for the development of a MenB vaccine, although I argue that the social support has been even more important for this vaccine, not only at the development stage but also to ensure wider policy adoption and public access.

How the MenB vaccine was supported by disease charities in the early 2000s – particularly the charity Meningitis Now – demonstrates the importance of a social drive. Professor Richard Moxon a leading, internationally renowned vaccinologist, who published on the complete genome MenB sequence and the identification of novel candidate vaccine antigens, recounted the early media interest in a vaccine in 2000 (Moxon 2021). He remembered a heading in the *Daily Mail* read, 'Meningitis: Breakthrough over vaccine that might have saved this little boy', with a picture of a 2-year-old who had died from meningitis (ibid., p. 181). Backing from meningitis charities , which included sharing stories of those affected by meningitis, helped drive forward the research, as they were willing to commit to the development of vaccines that were still some time away.

The MenB vaccine used in the United Kingdom, called Bexsero® was developed by Novartis (now GSK Biologicals). It was licensed by the European Medical Association (EMA) in January 2013 following extensive safety and effectiveness testing through 10 years of trials in the laboratory and with volunteers (Masignani, Pizza, and Moxon 2019).[2] On 3 December 2013, the vaccine was made available for private use in the United Kingdom at immunisation clinics and in some pharmacy groups.[3] When the vaccine

2 Bexsero® was also later licenced in the United States in 2015 (Brehony et al. 2015). A bivalent recombinant vaccine, the rLP2086 vaccine, Trumenba, had been developed by Pfizer and licenced by the FDA in the United States in 2014 (ibid.).

3 For example, in pharmacies Boots and Superdrug for £109 per dose, totalling £218–£327 per course. See: <https://healthclinics.superdrug.com/services/meningitis-b-vaccination> (accessed 31 July 2022).

was being evaluated by health economists, the price was at £75 a dose, with two to three doses per course required (Christensen et al. 2014). Bexsero® is unusual in that common side effects are reported but appear to be well tolerated. These include high rates of fever in infants, for which paracetamol is advised but even though the vaccine is quite reactogenic it has a high uptake and was so demanded by parents that a government ePetition was launched to extend its coverage from newborns to older children (Leston-Bandeira 2019). The parents behind the petition wanted the vaccine to be part of the schedule for older children stretching beyond the health authority rationale that the main burden of the disease was in young babies (with a peak around five to six months of age).

The ePetition and 'Beat It Now!' campaign

Advocacy for use of the MenB vaccine concentrated on the 'Beat It Now!' campaign by the charity Meningitis Now, which was established in 2013. The national charity that covers the whole of the United Kingdom was formed by the merger of two charities: Meningitis Trust and Meningitis UK (Millar et al. 2018). Meningitis Trust was originally established in 1982 as a parent-driven local support group raising money for meningitis research following an outbreak in Stroud, England, which later branched out to begin a 24-hour helpline offering nurse-led advice for questions about meningitis from both health professionals and the public (and still exists today) (BBC News 2013a). Meningitis UK was established in 1986 in Bristol, England, to fight meningitis and was set up by Steve Dayman, whose 14-month-old son Spencer had died of meningitis (Kirby 2022). Meningitis Now has grown substantially over the past decade, with success in fundraising and gaining public backing. Medical research, including supporting the development and introduction of vaccines against meningitis, has been a key part of their work, alongside awareness campaigns and providing practical, emotional, and financial assistance to people to rebuild their lives after illness. The charity had already played a role in funding the development and introduction in 1992 of a *Haemophilus influenzae* type b (Hib) vaccine, protecting against a bacterial infection which can cause meningitis (Meningitis Now n.d.). In 2013, the charity's United Kingdom-wide campaign began soon after the vaccine Bexsero® had been licensed in Europe. The 'Beat it Now!' campaign aimed to get the government to introduce the vaccine for free on the National Health System (NHS), as part of the national schedule across the United Kingdom.

The use of public petitions to show support for vaccination against meningitis had begun with an initial ePetition of 20,000 signatories demanding the introduction of the vaccine, delivered on 23 October 2013 to Downing Street (Warne 2013). On 14 January 2014, over 100 doctors, nurses, and scientists wrote a letter to Health Secretary Jeremy Hunt, urging him to introduce a vaccine for MenB. Eleven 'Young Ambassadors' delivered a petition with more than 36,000 signatures to Hunt and met with members of parliament (MPs) at Downing Street on 25 February 2014 (Meningitis Now n.d.). Meningitis Now ran a social media campaign in late 2014 targeting Hunt and calling for the early implementation of the MenB vaccine. Also important was asking MPs for their support and encouraging them to sign up to the Beat It Now! campaign (Image 3.1). Social media engagement reaching an estimated 2 million people online as well as regular stories in the mainstream media led to a high profile coverage (with for example Sue Davis, the chief executive of the charity, telephoning into Nick Clegg's LBC radio show and asking why the vaccine was taking so long). The charity campaigned for over a year, and much of the focus of the ongoing advocacy was on the fear and needless devastation caused by the disease, portrayed through the accounts of families affected, as Stroud MP Neil Carmichael relayed:

> Meningitis is unpredictable and is still the disease feared most by parents. Vaccines have made a huge impact on cases but I was shocked to hear that it still affects thousands of people every year. (Warne 2013)

The first step after achieving public and political visibility was to start the policy process for change. The Joint Committee on Vaccination and Immunisation (JCVI) plays an influential role in any recommendation for government policy. This expert advisory committee advises United Kingdom Health Department about immunisation on the basis of the safety, efficacy, and cost-effectiveness of vaccines. On 21 March 2014, the

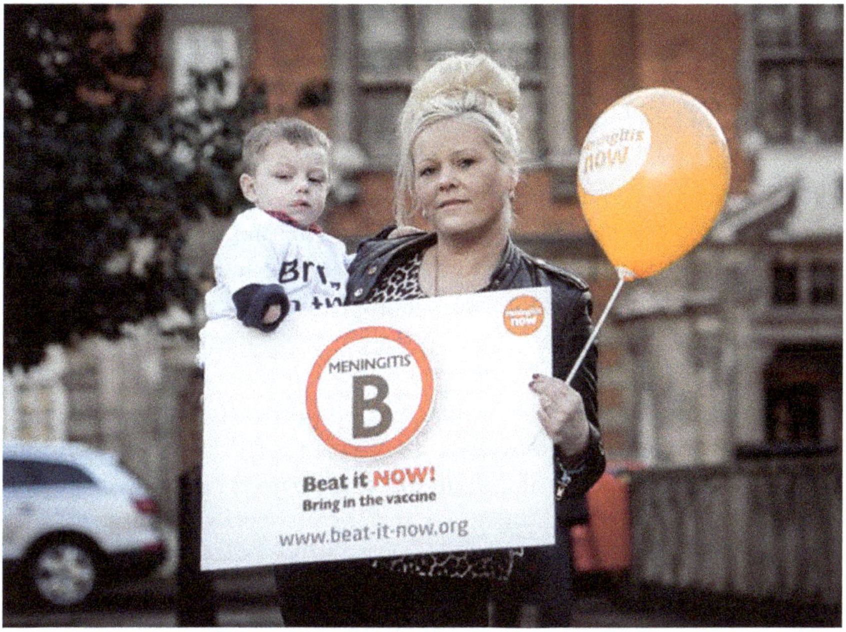
MENINGITIS
B
Beat it NOW!
Bring in the vaccine
www.beat-it-now.org

Image 3.1 'Beat It Now!' campaign poster.

With permission from Meningitis Now. 2015. <https://www.meningitisnow.org/meningitis-now-stories/campaigns/beat-it-now/>

JCVI recommended the vaccine be introduced into the national schedule (Meningitis Now n.d.). In November 2014, Meningitis Now and MPs met at the House of Commons with an update on the vaccine negotiations requested at Prime Minister's Questions (a weekly Parliament session where the prime minister answers questions from MPs). Successful negotiations were announced on 29 March 2015, and the vaccine was introduced into the national schedule in September that year. After the introduction of the vaccine, Meningitis Now did not stop their advocacy work. On 2 November 2015, the charity wrote to Jeremy Hunt and the Department of Health to extend the vaccine to all children in every family where there had been a case of meningitis. They also asked general practitioners (GPs) to support the wider rollout. Their concentration was on broadening the access to the MenB vaccine.

In 2016, a second ePetition in the United Kingdom aimed to extend vaccine provision of the MenB vaccine to older children over 12 months, which was limited to be given only to babies at two and four months old, followed by a booster at 12 months as part of a nationwide campaign (Meningitis Now n.d.). On 14 February 2016, the death of two-year-old Faye Burdett, whose death from MenB was covered widely in the press, triggered an emotional response to the issue of meningitis and the ePetition in association (Image 3.2). The family released a powerful image of their daughter taken shortly before she died, seriously ill in hospital, hooked up to many tubes with blood blotches all over her body and the pictures made national headlines.

The ePetition was eventually signed by 823,341 people. At the time, it was the largest parliamentary petition and following two oral evidence sessions was debated in the House of Commons, as happens for any ePetition with over 100,000 signatures (Watson 2020). The first parliamentary evidence

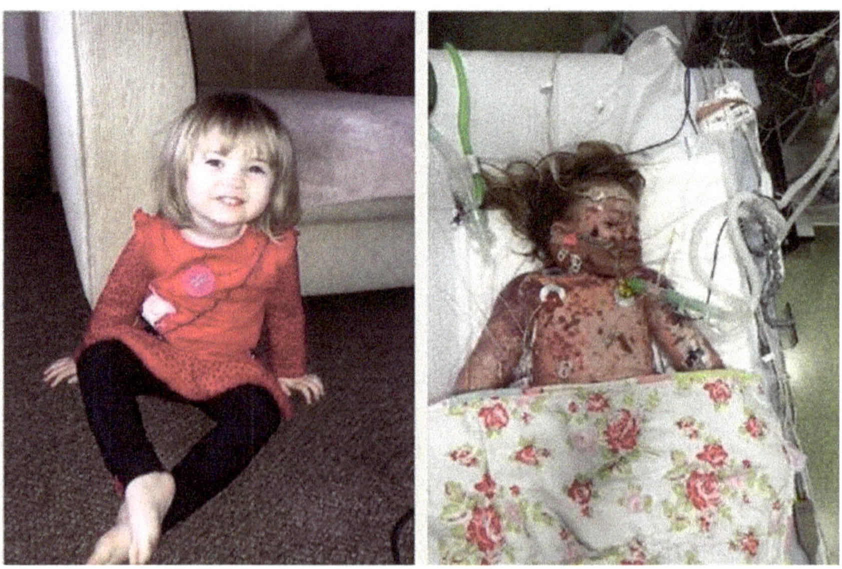

Image 3.2 Faye Burdett.

With permission from Meningitis Now. 2016. <https://meningitisnow.dedicationpage.org/virtualgarden/Dedications/24552>

session was held in March 2016 for families affected and the second was for experts and professional organisations at the Parliamentary Petitions Committee and Health Committee. In addition, that year, an upsurge in demand led to a shortage of the MenB vaccine in private clinics, with the data showing that the vaccine was already having an impact in cases for vaccine-eligible children within 10 months of the programme starting. However, on 14 June government health advisers rejected the ePetition call for children up to two years old to be given the MenB vaccine based on the cost and lack of supply. A year later, Jenny and Neil Burdett expressed their disappointment at the lack of progress for an extension of the age eligibility on the first anniversary of their daughter Faye's death.

While unsuccessful at the time, the ePetition still showed a strong public vaccine support. The distinct grouping being represented included the affected charities and parents, the originators of the petition being Jenny and Neil Burdett (from Maidstone in the South) and another parent, Lee Booth (based in the Northeast). Booth had been concerned about his daughter being too old to have the free access to the vaccine and wanted it to be more widely available to the public. The meningitis charities, particularly Meningitis Now, had been campaigning a long time for a MenB vaccine to be developed and then be on the national schedule. The ePetition to extend the age eligibility generated most of the publicity through a Facebook group and was linked to other Facebook groups, including one with mothers who had all had children in the same month. One of those had been Jenny Burdett, whose daughter Faye had contracted MenB and was in a serious condition in hospital at the time.

When the ePetition aims were rejected, it was a knock-back for advocates who wanted the vaccine to be available more widely, and showed a limit to public support of vaccination in the face of arguments grounded on measurement and evidence-based logic. Other factors of public health intervention were considered, including the opportunity cost of limited resources, the difference an intervention makes on disease burden, and the toleration of the public to accept more vaccines. The JCVI slightly amended their advice since the House of Commons debate and have conceded that MenB would be cost-effective at a very low price for children up to the age of 2 years instead of one year (Barber 2016), but it is unlikely to be sold at such a price. No change to the national schedule was made for a catch-up programme for older children because, on balance, it was not cost-effective.

Nevertheless, while the ePetition was unsuccessful, it put pressure on the government from MPs and the public. As political scientist Cristina Leston-Bandeira has found, although the majority of ePetitions to the United Kingdom Parliament are rejected and only a small proportion lead to action, they 'play an important role' in scrutinising the government and facilitating public campaigning and engagement (2019b, p. 1). In the case of the MenB ePetition, an element of public engagement was sustained through the regular email updates sent to signatories, including links to relevant material. There was also a 'gathering evidence' function, through the oral evidence sessions held by the Petitions Committee with four panels, which included both affected families and experts used to inform the debate. Ultimately, the government did resolve to follow up on the issue through regular correspondence with the Department of Health and was compelled to react in some way (ibid.). The health minister Jane Ellison announced she was launching a national awareness campaign about the symptoms of meningitis, and there is now an ongoing review of the cost-effectiveness methodology for immunisation (Department of Health and Social Care Media Centre 2016). More widely, it has helped generate publicity for the vaccination and increased awareness of meningitis. In 2018, the government was summoned to give new evidence to the committee, and it published a very delayed report. The evidence session was described as 'tense', and the minister said that pressure from the committee had prompted the report's publication (2019, p. 21).

While the focus of policy change has often been on the centres of policy power, online activity surrounding the ePetition also means it has had a wider public impact. However, this example of wider availability and coverage of vaccination being sought, only referred to a specific vaccine, rather than an activist group supporting all vaccination and reducing all vaccine-preventable disease deaths. Support was mainly driven by impacted parents and disease charities; but importantly, many of those in the constituency made reference to the importance of and respect towards science and evidence. What then does the MenB ePetition say about the shape of pro-vaccine support? The means taken for action was through a public participatory route arguing for policy change. It is because vaccination is endorsed by public policy that this route is attractive. In the United Kingdom, the extension of vaccine provision did not particularly tread into anti-vaccine territory, especially in relation to a disease that many parents are afraid of. It directly targeted the intricacies of the national schedule and technical advice of the JCVI. Therefore, the specificity of the campaign appears to have suited both those who are supportive or critical of vaccination (by not involving them in any meaningful way).

The United Kingdom was to be the first country in the world to introduce the MenB vaccine into its routine vaccination schedule and results have influenced other countries' decisions to include the vaccine (Jackson et al. 2017). Concerning other vaccines against meningitis in the United Kingdom, teenagers aged 13–14 (school year nine) and students going to university or college for the first time are currently being offered the MenACWY vaccine,[4] called Nimenrix (Vaccine Knowledge, n.d.). These are the groups most likely to carry and spread the bacteria. Even though, historically, the United Kingdom had been lagging behind in introducing new vaccines; by the 1990s it had adopted new vaccines against Hib and pneumococcus early, partly because these vaccines had their first population-level assessment there (Miles 2023). The United Kingdom led the world in co-developing the MenC vaccine (NmCV) with three manufacturers, which was able to provide long-term protection and could be used for babies and young children, and was also the first country in the world to introduce it in 1999 (Wise 1999). Other countries then initiated major vaccination campaigns against meningitis, such as the Dutch campaign for universal vaccination against infections with group C meningococci and pneumococci, offered to children older than 12 months. This decision followed an increase in the number of serotyped cases of MenC in the Netherlands, which had risen from 86 in 1999 to 275 in 2001 (Esveld 2002). Outbreaks that had already occurred were being controlled by local vaccination campaigns, and many parents had their children immunised

4 The quadrivalent (A, C, Y, and W) meningococcal conjugate vaccines were licensed in 2009 (Brady et al. 2011).

early at their own expense, with the vaccination campaign reportedly being the largest in Dutch history at the time.

The United Kingdom has remained an example of meningitis advocacy, but the possibilities of public support should be viewed on a wider scale for global health. The highest burden of disease is still in the meningitis belt of sub-Saharan Africa, despite the positive impact of the MenA vaccine there. It is an issue of health equity that the disease burden and access to vaccines is most problematic in sub-Saharan Africa, and not Western Europe. Across the meningitis belt that covers 26 countries from Senegal in the west to Ethiopia in the east, each year approximately 30,000 cases are reported (WHO n.d.). A vaccine for MenA was rolled out in 2010 through mass preventive immunisation campaigns in the meningitis belt. The MenAfriVac® vaccine,[5] was developed in 2010 through a partnership between World Health Organization (WHO), PATH, and Serum Institute of India Pvt. Ltd (SIIPL) and available in sub-Saharan Africa since 2017 onwards (Laforce et al. 2017).[6] The WHO has set a roadmap to defeat meningitis by 2030 in what has been described as 'an ambitious target' (Greenwood, Sow, and Preziosi 2021), and in July 2023, MenFive® against serogroups A, C, W, X, and Y achieved pre-qualification with the WHO to protect against the five predominant causes of meningococcal meningitis in Africa (PATH 2023).[7]

5 A monovalent group A meningococcal conjugate vaccine (NmCV-A).

6 As a result of Meningitis Vaccine Project (MVP), a Gates Foundation funded partnership.

7 A pentavalent NmCV developed by SIIPL and PATH with funding from the UK government's Foreign, Commonwealth and Development Office. Prequalification is the WHO approval for safety and effectiveness.

Measles and pertussis – pro-vaccine activism

Next, I provide examples of how activism differs within different country contexts in the political economy of healthcare. While public petitions and the advocacy work of charities in the meningitis example may be a more an established route to pursue an interest-based cause, activism takes on various forms depending on the context. Comparing case studies of pro-vaccine activism across India, Australia, and the United States, the societal response to childhood diseases (namely measles and pertussis that have had a recent resurgence) becomes apparent. India exemplifies the everyday work of civil society actors to promote vaccination with partnerships through the media, alongside individual doctors, and their activities implemented at local levels to build confidence.[8] In Australia and the United States, I document two concerted citizen-led campaigns of pro-vaccine activism, with the Australian case showing a combination of grassroots organisation and media engagement, and the American case bringing activism to the political stage.[9] I examine the types of practices and strategies employed by activists to voice their support of vaccination and discuss the means, messages, and motivations of pro-vaccine activism.

Pro-vaccine support in India

The pro-vaccine public in India follows a typical pattern seen in many countries. What can be observed are actors such as the mainstream media working alongside government and with other policy interventions. However, the media has also offered a push-back when interventions

8 I rely on the research I provided for a joint paper about vaccination narratives (Vanderslott et al. 2022).

9 I first outlined these case studies in depth through the following paper: 'Exploring the meaning of pro-vaccine activism across two countries' (Vanderslott 2019). I drew on qualitative research (university ethical approval: R50658/RE001).

are heavy-handed and have other adverse effects, especially for marginalised populations (a point discussed later). As often, the balance between a public health intervention and the imposition of other restrictions or unintended consequences is a continued policy challenge. Such contradictions have become apparent in India, which is a leading producer and exporter of vaccines, but still holds a large share of the world's unimmunised children and vaccine-preventable childhood diseases, with measles and rubella remaining endemic. Measles outbreaks kill nearly 50,000 children each year in India, amounting to over one-third of global measles deaths, while rubella infection causes birth defects in almost 40,000 children annually (WHO 2019a). Since 1985, the Indian Ministry of Health and Family Welfare has overseen a Universal Immunisation Programme (UIP) with support from international institutions such as the WHO (Lahariya 2014). The high number of preventable deaths and disabilities is why the WHO and the Indian government set a target for the elimination of measles and control of rubella before 2020 (Vaidya et al. 2016).

When India adopted the Expanded Programme on Immunization (EPI) in 1978, the measles vaccine was not included, as measles was believed to not be a widespread problem at the time (Jacob John and Verghese 2011). The government has since integrated the measles and rubella (MR) vaccine into the national schedule, free of cost, starting with a campaign run by the Union Health Ministry of vaccinating in the states of Tamil Nadu, Karnataka, and Goa, and the union territories (UTs) of Lakshadweep and Puducherry. A phased rollout beginning with a limited number of states and territories was seen to be more manageable. This state-sponsored MR mass vaccination drive ran from 2017 to 2018. The wider global campaign also encompassed ten other WHO South-East Asia Region member countries who were aiming to eliminate measles and rubella (Vaidya et al. 2016). The first phase was carried out in schools, community centres, and health facilities. As a result, more than 33 million children were vaccinated, and the campaign was initially a success, reaching out to 97 per cent of the intended age group (Kaul 2017). On the ground, health promoters got involved in raising awareness about the campaign. In one example, a pharmacist shared a cartoon of a family, which went viral on local WhatsApp groups (Raison

2017). The cartoon (see Image 3.3), which was not part of the official campaign, shows a family being vaccinated and included an affirming message about the campaign, written in the local Pahari language.

As the campaign moved to the second phase in August 2017, it scaled up its aim to vaccinate 41 million children (aged from 9 months to 15 years) across a total of eight states and UTs: Andhra Pradesh, Chandigarh, Dadra and Nagar Haveli, Daman and Diu, Himachal Pradesh, Kerala, Telangana, and Uttarakhand. The bar was set high as one of the biggest worldwide vaccination campaigns and after its completion the MR vaccine would replace the measles-only vaccine in routine immunisation. In recognising the central role of the media, ahead of the second phase launch, a 'Regional Media Workshop' was held by the Ministry of Health and Family Welfare, in association with the United Nations International Children's Emergency

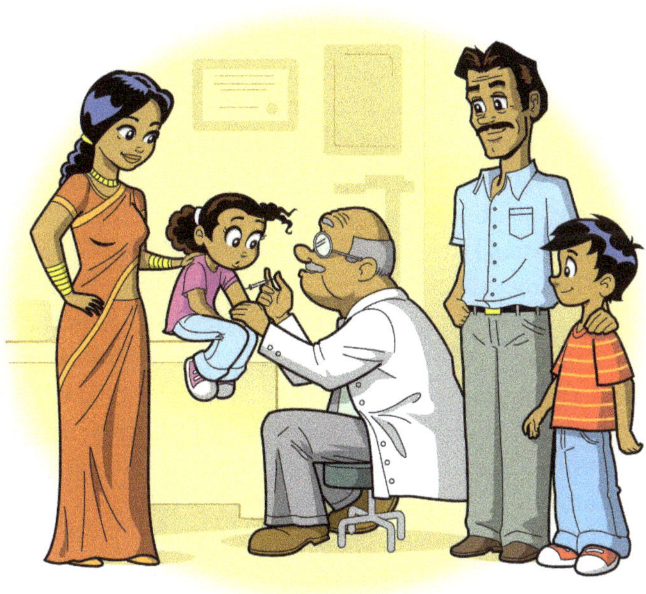

Image 3.3 Measles-rubella campaign cartoon.

Kenny Kiernan in Raison (2017).

Fund (UNICEF) and the WHO alongside key media partners. The motivation to engage with the media as a critical stakeholder was part of an effort to 'create trust in vaccines and address myths around immunisation to ensure every child in the country gets a fair start' (*Hindu* 2017). The mainstream mostly newspaper and broadcast media had a long-standing position of influence in Indian vaccination policies since the fight against polio (Jeffery and Jeffery 2011).

A concentration on the awareness and acceptance of vaccination, however, further discounts issues that have often been identified as problems with the 'supply side'. This is a lack of investment in immunisation services and supply chain issues getting from vaccine production to deployment. The 'demand side' has gained increased attention and is sought to be influenced through media engagement. Slow vaccine acceptance rooted in ignorant anti-vaccine beliefs is blamed for poor vaccine coverage, and so the media is viewed as an important ally to overcome this (Lahariya 2014). The *Hindustan Times* expressed in their 2019 headline: 'Vaccines save lives, ignorance jeopardises them', stating: 'Rumours, falsehoods and blatant fabrications about the side effects of vaccination spread faster than the common cold' (Sharma 2019). The 'Muslim opposition' to the MR vaccination was identified in news reports early on. This characterisation of opposition was based on a portrayal of age-old prejudices which deemed immunisation as un-Islamic. One headline, in a leading news channel, read: 'Vaccination Drive Extended After Hitting a Wall in Muslim Pockets' (Tripathi 2017) (Image 3.4). The story described how 'anti-vaxxers' were 'using a statement by Union Minister of State Kiren Rijiju to further their propaganda against the very idea of vaccination' via misinformation on WhatsApp groups, claiming that the vaccine was an imported and untried one, causing impotency and autism (ibid.). Reports continued to reference how paranoia about vaccines had been a long-standing problem in India ever since the Pulse Polio campaign (Jayarajan 2020) (Image 3.5).

The Pulse Polio campaign, launched in 1995, was a public health intervention where Muslims were described to be at the 'sharp end' in being targeted and blamed for low vaccine uptake (Jeffery and Jeffery 2011). Despite ultimately being a success, the campaign was seen as problematic and biased. Poor communication about the need for repeated vaccination,

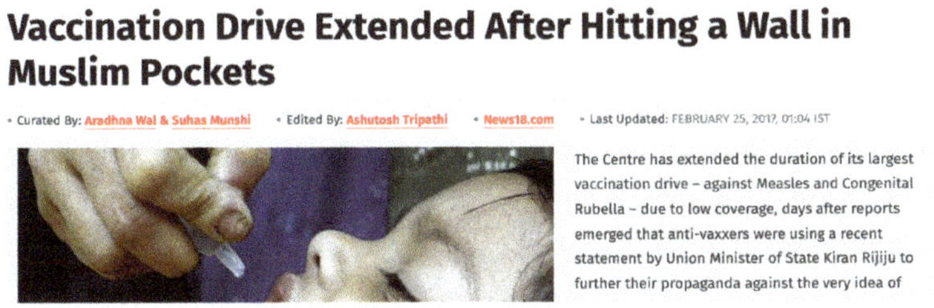

Vaccination Drive Extended After Hitting a Wall in Muslim Pockets

• Curated By: Aradhna Wal & Suhas Munshi • Edited By: Ashutosh Tripathi • News18.com • Last Updated: FEBRUARY 25, 2017, 01:04 IST

The Centre has extended the duration of its largest vaccination drive – against Measles and Congenital Rubella – due to low coverage, days after reports emerged that anti-vaxxers were using a recent statement by Union Minister of State Kiran Rijiju to further their propaganda against the very idea of

Image 3.4 News18 headline about measles and rubella vaccination drive.

<https://www.news18.com/news/india/vaccination-drive-extended-as-campaign-hits-propaganda-wall-in-muslim-pockets-1352897.html>

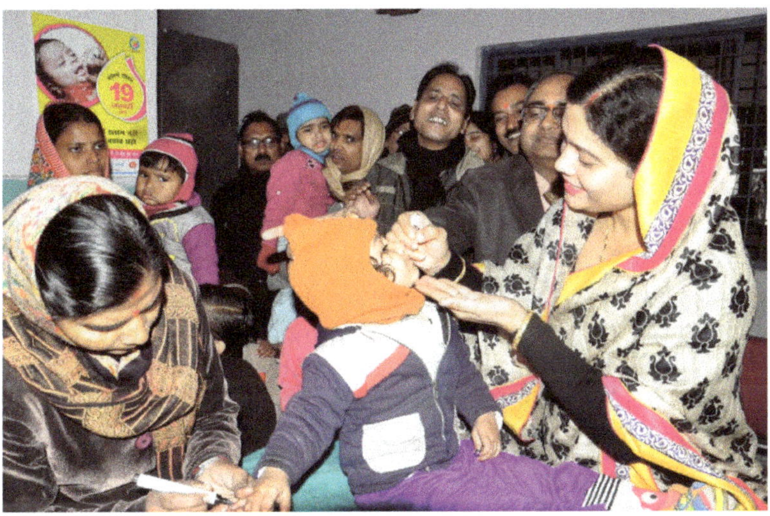

Image 3.5 'Pulse Polio' campaign in Delhi.

The Delhi government campaign was called Polio Ravivar (Polio Sunday). Wikimedia Commons/

as well as about the circulation of poliovirus through open defecation, monsoons, and inadequate water treatment, led to parents being sceptical about whether the vaccine worked (Hussain et al. 2012). The absence of other free healthcare also raised suspicions and rumours that the vaccine caused infertility. Therefore, there were practical and supply-side reasons for a lack of public confidence, not captured in a demand-side view of vaccine hesitancy rooted in ignorance.

As India is a Hindu-majority country where Muslims form a significant minority, community membership and identity are central to understanding the concerns of vaccinating publics. Lower vaccine coverage among religious minorities is frequently presented as a threat to the immunity of the nation-state, which pits the minority groups against nationalist ideals (Kasstan 2019). Within this mix, intra- and interfaith divisions are compounded by politics and other local constituencies that contribute to views on vaccination. In addition, the circulation of myths and rumours are reflective of anxieties and concerns, while community leaders are sometimes promoters or antagonists of public health messaging. These minority vs state issues are evident both through public health programmes and in the responses to these programmes. The issue at hand may appear to be about vaccine hesitancy based on religious beliefs, but it also provides insight into the will of the government to have compliance, and the resistance of minority publics. As anthropologist Ben Kasstan points out, state attempts to enforce vaccination policies, 'play into entrenched minority-state tensions' (2019, p. 2).

Similar to the reasons for unease regarding polio vaccination, low uptake for the MR vaccine has also been explained by focusing blame on the Muslim sector of the population – rather than, for instance, by addressing a history of discriminatory treatment in health services. Furthermore, the opposition to the MR vaccine took on a political dimension as a way to voice dissatisfaction with and signal distrust towards the ruling Bharatiya Janata Party (BJP). Elected in 2014, the BJP has been accused of a 'Hindu-first agenda' to the detriment of Muslims in India and attacks on minorities, which has increased to be more systematic and banal (Anderson and Jaffrelot 2018). A 35-year-old from Kondotty, directly addressing Prime Minister Modi, exemplified the anti-government sentiment: 'This is Modi-RSS vaccine. You are doing this to control our population. Please go away. I will not allow my children to be vaccinated' (Nair 2017). RSS stands for Rashtriya Swayamsevak Sangh, a right-wing Hindu nationalist organisation that operates as a volunteer paramilitary group.

Those opposing the vaccination were referred to as 'trolls', exemplified by such headlines as 'Tamil Nadu government to take on trolls against Measles-Rubella vaccine drive' (Jane 2017). The state government warned 'trolls' that they could face criminal action for spreading 'canards' (unfounded rumours or stories) about the vaccination drive, and the vaccination campaign was extended due to low coverage. Therefore, the government's most negative reference to the vaccinating public was directed at those who spread misinformation such as traditional healers who were offering explanations to a suspicious public. The government worried about the spread of misinformation, which is why they took a strong stance against those disrupting a high-profile, politically important campaign.

The individual states and UTs worked on a response, with the advocacy of doctors proving instrumental. Doctors enlisted their students to help, worked with district health officers, as well as with writers, and journalists, and broadcast radio programmes to communicate about the benefits of immunisation – even using magicians to bust myths (Tripathi 2017). In Tamil Nadu, a group of doctors also took legal means to lodge a formal complaint via the Chief Minister's Grievance Cell against a Coimbatore-based 'healer' (Jane 2017) who had claimed in messages circulated on social media and instant messaging platforms that the vaccine contained disease-causing organisms. The interventions were effective, and India continues to make progress towards measles elimination and rubella control. By July 2018, 92 million children had been successfully vaccinated, edging closer to the target to cover 405 million children (WHO 2019a). In 2022, India launched the Intensified Mission Indradhanush (IMI) 4.0 to achieve the goal of full universal immunisation coverage for 90 per cent of the population and moving towards MR elimination (WHO 2022).

Pro-vaccine activism in Australia and the United States

In other countries, citizen support for vaccination has been more overt, bringing an activist dimension towards decision making in government and the media. Next, I provide two case studies as prominent examples of such overt support.[10] In both cases, activism is directed at those opposed to vaccination or at under-vaccinating communities. These are studies of highly visible pro-vaccine activism, with oppositional counteractivities in favour of vaccination in Australia, and issue-based advocacy as part of a political alliance in the United States, during measles and pertussis outbreaks. At this citizen level, pro-vaccine activism has similarities to the Indian case in reinforcing the mainstream view and countering digression from it. Two groups, Vaccinate California in the United States and Stop the AVN (SAVN) in Australia, offer insight into how pro-vaccine activism had impact.[11] The focus in Australia comes from a pro-science stance, where mainstream scientific consensus is supported, and includes 'sceptics' against pseudoscience directly opposing vaccine-critical groups. In the United States, the focus takes the form of an issue-specific campaign

10 Drawn from an earlier study with 25 semi-structured interviews gathering information on activist activities over 8 months from June 2017 to February 2018 (Vanderslott 2019).

11 Interviewee selection began with a core set of founders, members, and supporters of both groups, followed by snowball sampling of a second set of actors in their immediate networks. The Vaccinate California case study included nine interviews with founders, policy officials, academics, and non-government organisation workers, along with eight interviews with local health authorities in California, which were done face-to-face. The SAVN case study included eight interviews with SAVN members based in Australia, as well as with health authorities, academics, and groups influenced. Interviews took place via video call due to the geographic distance between interviewees and took on average 70 minutes, with some email correspondence to share material and for further discussion. Interviewees signed formal consent with an anonymisation option.

that has arisen from existing pro-vaccine parent blogs and discussion groups pushing for policy change rather than public confrontation.

Pro-vaccine activist groups here take one of two distinct forms: collectively minded, parent-based groups fostered via mainstream political actors; or pro-science and anti-pseudoscience movements that directly oppose anti-vaccine views and activity.[12] I showcase the impact of active civil society organisation to promote vaccination by countering anti-vaccine groups and influencing changes in policy and media representation. Using semi-structured interviews I developed a multilayered depiction of the formation and strategies of both groups. My questions centred around how interviewees viewed themselves as being 'pro-vaccine': what drove such views; the internal structure and history of their organisation, their aims and activities; how that related to other groups and institutions, broader societal implications of their actions, and the regional and country context. I was aware that the pro-vaccine activists could find it socially desirable to tone down views (Kuran 1995). This came across through dismissiveness towards opposing views (i.e. 'it is not worth trying to change their minds'). After completing the interviews, I concentrated on identifying 'storylines' of policy processes, public engagement over time, and how actors developed versions of a story (Hajer 2009). The storylines that became apparent included the 'triggers' for their actions, which was the 2015 measles outbreak for Vaccinate California and the treatment of parents (the McCafferys) in the case of SAVN.

I also drew upon a variety of documentary sources, including the activist groups' materials (websites, social media sites, and court transcripts), the state archives (on Senate Bill SB 277 to ban non-medical exemptions to vaccination), materials obtained through interviews (reports and presentations), media accounts accessed through the LexisNexis database, and newspaper archives (using keyword searches of: Vaccinate California, SB 277, SAVN, AVN). The themes that came out concentrated on the origins

12 In addition, I interviewed five academics involved with the groups, to gain perspective on how those researching controversial topics can be drawn into the debate (Scott, Richards, and Martin 1990). The academics reported hostile behaviour from actors they were critical of.

of the groups and their reasons for forming (external events, values, and norms), main motivations (what they hoped to achieve and measurement of success), situation in the policy and media context, and comparisons to other group or country contexts.[13]

Vaccinate California and SAVN

In Australia, pro-vaccine activism has focused on resisting a vaccine-critical group established in 1994 by parent Meryl Dorey, originally called the Australian Vaccination Network, renamed the Australian Vaccination-Skeptics Network and then the Australian Vaccination-Risks Network (AVN). Stop the AVN (SAVN) was formed in 2009 with the explicit aim to shut down the AVN. Through direct confrontation, SAVN has dramatically limited AVN activities and is likely to continue opposing the AVN and similar groups and individuals. In comparison, the United States has witnessed a less confrontational, more issue-specific campaign to boost child vaccination in California. The focus was enacting a particular policy (California Senate Bill SB 277) and legal change, rather than wider societal or ideational change, and its activities more or less ceased after the bill was successfully passed.

Creating a shared identity to attract new supporters and also easily convey the values of the groups was important and is reflected in their branding. SAVN states its aim in explicit terms through the assertive stop-sign imagery of their logo (Image 3.6). The AVN logo, meanwhile, shows its need to portray care for babies and children (Image 3.7). The logo of another Australian pro-vaccine group, the Northern Rivers Vaccination Supporters (NRVS), takes a similar stance in depicting a large, happy family

13 The methodological limitations were largely due to observing people and events outside the country context and not in real time. As a result, some contextual country points may have been missed, including related discussions happening at that time. The selection of two cases is also limited in not depicting pro-vaccine activism widely.

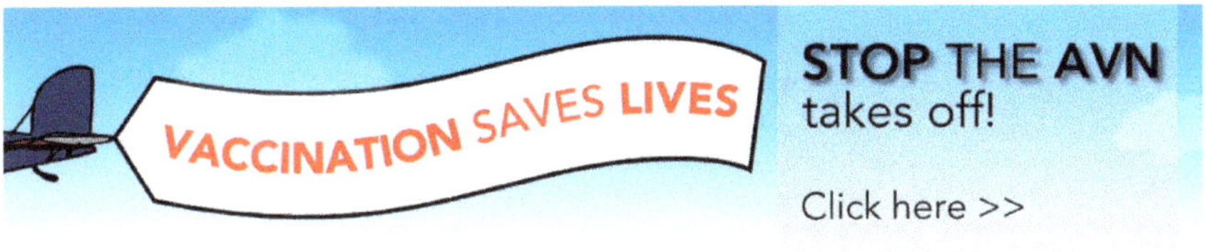

Image 3.6 Stop the AVN (SAVN) logo.
<https://stopavn.com/>

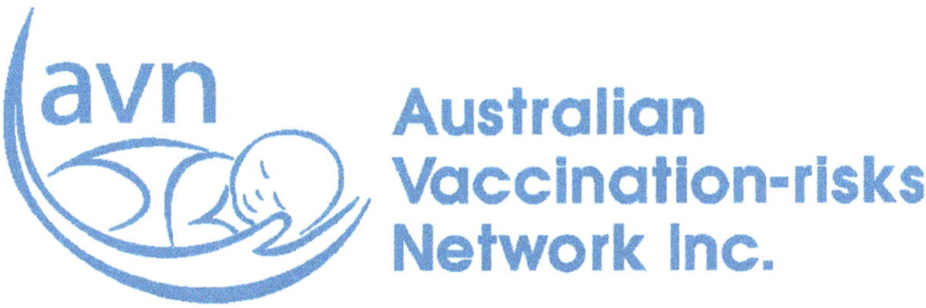

Image 3.7 Australian Vaccination-Risks Network (AVN) logo.
<https://avn.org.au/>

(Image 3.8). The focus here may be on the collective rather than the individual; they are both similar in also portraying hands as a symbol of caring.

In the United States, the 2015 Disneyland measles outbreak in Orange County, California, brought the issue of vaccination to the forefront in the state. The major disruption caused was described by law professor Dorit Reiss: 'Cases from the measles Disneyland outbreak went to 170 [...] And we exported it to 16 additional states, to Mexico, and to Canada. California would rather be known as an exporter of movies and avocado than of measles' (Reiss, interview with author, 2017). Prior to 2015, California had been called an 'epicenter of vaccine refusal' (Dr Blaise Congeni, quoted in Khimm 2010) – a claim that may have been exaggerated at the time but nonetheless demonstrates how the blame for the outbreak was pointed squarely at those who refused vaccination. As Hausmann notes, what developed from 2004 onwards was a 'trend of arguing against vaccine skeptics

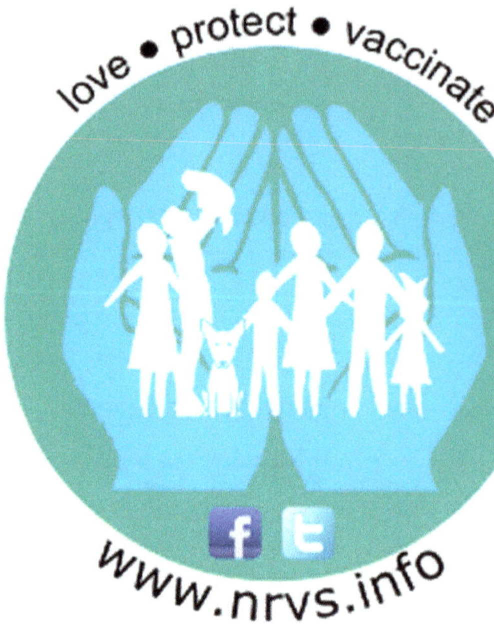

Image 3.8 Northern Rivers Vaccination Supporters (NRVS) logo.
<https://nrvs.info/>

and for the value of vaccination' (2019a, pp. 41–2). Similarly, as Brunson and Sobo describe, although public debates about vaccination emphasise polarities which are rarely accurate and mostly stereotypical, this still points to how 'polarization feeds on itself, further strengthening the perception of a divide' (2017, p. 46).

The incident caused pro-vaccine parents to reinforce their position. Journalist Tara Haelle describes how this created a unique situation with pro-vaccine parents spurred into action by a 'direct threat to their children' (Milken Institute School of Public Health 2015). Doctors reported how some parents did not want to be in the same waiting room as unvaccinated families, a change in tone described by this father: 'Before, I thought, "If you think your child will become autistic, fine". But now they're pushing their beliefs on everybody, and I feel differently' (Healy and Paulson 2015). Reiss also spoke of her experience as a social media commentator: 'After the Disneyland outbreak, you suddenly saw a dramatic growth in people speaking on the pro-vaccine side. And many of them were people that never were active before' (interview with author, 2017).

In California, pro-vaccine groups have existed for some time. California, like all other states, has an 'immunization coalition' comprised of community partners interested in improving vaccination provision and uptake. There are parent-led pro-vaccine groups present on a national level (including 'Voices for Vaccines' and 'Moms Who Vax'). A 'deficit model of public understanding', wherein a lack of information about vaccination fuels incorrect and negative views, has been a driving approach behind communication campaigns, but there is growing recognition that the model is flawed (Leach and Fairhead 2007). Simply supplying better and more information about vaccines is an insufficient strategy, and more participatory engagement is thought to be needed. The way that publics come to form a view on vaccination is changing, and according to Christine Vara, editor of the 'Vaccinate Your Family' Facebook page and the blog 'A Shot of Prevention', social media is playing a bigger role: 'Things were being said and there was nobody really there to say, "Whoa, wait a minute, that's not really how it is"' (interview with author, 2017). These groups aim to reach out to vaccine-hesitant parents and convince them to vaccinate, or support healthcare workers to engage in conversations with parents through the use of vaccination stories and educational materials. The effort to increase vaccination rates is largely limited to discussing vaccine facts.

Some parents thought the situation needed solving through legislation. California State Senators Dr Richard Pan and Ben Allen authored Senate Bill SB 277 to remove non-medical exemptions for vaccination requirements. Vaccination is mandatory in all states to attend public school, state-licensed childcare, family day care and developmental centres, along with some private institutions in the United States (Orenstein and Hinman 1999). However, all states allow for medical exemptions, and two at the time (Mississippi and West Virginia) did not allow for any other types of exemptions (i.e. on philosophical, personal, or religious grounds). The senators were already supportive figures: Pan, a paediatrician, had experienced a measles outbreak in Philadelphia and passed Assembly Bill AB 2109 in 2012 to make religious and philosophical exemptions harder to obtain, while Allen's father was a polio survivor. Both wanted to take action but felt it was impossible without a strong parental push to convince the wider public and Senate; a constituency needed to be built. The senators made calls to parent groups on social media, to which four mothers responded, and Vaccinate California was formed in 2015 to co-sponsor SB 277 (Vaccinate California n.d.) (Image 3.9).

The Vaccinate California cofounders were four closely connected mothers: full-time mother and ex-lawyer Leah Russin, designer Hannah Nery, technology and finance analyst Renne Diresta, and full-time mother and former public relations worker Jennifer Wonnacott – all with skillsets contributing to particular aspects of the group's activities (Vaccinate California n.d.). They went on to recruit 20–30 other supporters, assigning tasks to each depending on their strengths. Vaccinate California did not

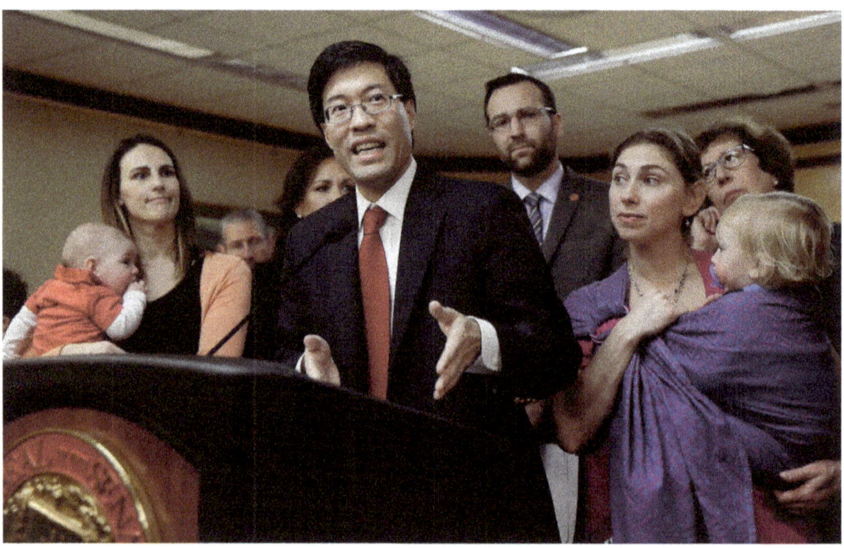

Image 3.9 Senators with Vaccinate California members.
<https://sd26.senate.ca.gov/photo-gallery>

engage directly with vaccine-hesitant or vaccine-refusing parents, who were directed to other resources. Their baseline position was: 'The vast majority agree with vaccination. They vaccinate and go about their business' (Russin, interview with author, 2017). The mission was to turn 'quiet pro-vaccine parents' into 'noisy pro-vaccine parents' and generate an alternative to the loud anti-vaxxer as described by cofounder Renee DiResta (2017): 'The anti-vaxx movement is well-organized, it's well-funded, and it's media-savvy [...] Legislators are only hearing from the passionate minority.' Vaccinate California made a point of not arguing about vaccine science, autism, or conspiracy theories but responded to discussion about parental rights and choice. They argued that immunocompromised children's right to health and education trumps the right of parents to ignore science, as Russin's testimony before the Senate Judiciary Committee demonstrates: 'We have the right not to have our children endangered at school by preventable disease. There are parents who disagree with me [...] But their decision not only jeopardizes the health and safety of their children, it puts my child at risk and that is unfair' (Whatthefolly 2015).

Vaccinate California mainly put forward their views through Facebook, bringing together dozens of pro-vaccine parenting groups. Russin found that many had legitimate questions (e.g. about vaccination schedules) but were 'jumped on' by anti-vaxxers before anyone else could answer. Twitter, according to Russin, attracted the more 'tin-foil-hat types' not worthy of engagement. Mainstream media coverage, however, proved problematic: 'Telling the story of Vaccinate California is not as interesting as an anti-vax one [...] the news media think they are repeating fact, but they write about conflict' (Russin, interview with author, 2017). Through their online presence, they collected 32,770 signatures supporting the Senate Bill, which they delivered to the senators, and were supported by figures such as a 6-year-old Californian boy suffering from leukaemia named Rhett Krawitt, who made a personal appeal for stronger policies to protect the immunocompromised (Change.org n.d.). Gaining traction through Facebook and ePetitions, Vaccinate California provided parental support and legitimacy to the Senate Bill. By 2016, SB 277 came into force, removing non-medical exemptions in California. However, conflict is not dispelled completely, as protests and lawsuits still continued from those opposing the bill (Sisson

2016). Vaccinate California addressed falling vaccination rates and consequent disease outbreak with a solution sought primarily through policy and legal means.

In Australia, by contrast, SAVN was reacting to the treatment of a bereaved family by a vaccine-critical group and saw the shutdown of that particular group as its main goal. The event that sparked SAVN was the death of 4-week-old Dana McCaffery due to pertussis (whooping cough). The day before the funeral, the media reported that the president of the AVN, Meryl Dorey, had tried to obtain Dana's medical records (Hansen 2013a). Although Dorey contends that she did not, she does assert she wanted proof of death from pertussis and questioned the finger-pointing at those opposed to vaccination: 'To my mind, an entire community of conscientious objectors were being victimised by the government and the media and being blamed for the death of a child who was too young to be vaccinated' (Dorey, n.d.).

The McCafferys established a website and Facebook page, telling Dana's story as an educational tool for vaccination (Hansen 2013a). They saw it as a community service in order to raise awareness of the importance of pertussis boosters (where an extra dose of the vaccine is received during pregnancy). They subsequently received a letter, including AVN pamphlets, to their home address, 'telling them they should have just stayed at home and breastfed the baby' (ibid.). Also, on the Australian national television programme ABC 7.30 Report, the McCafferys and Dorey appeared together speaking about pertussis vaccination. After it aired, Dorey encouraged her subscribers to complain to ABC about the show's editing, and posted on the McCafferys' website questioning vaccines. Andrew McDonald, a regular on AVN forums, even sent an email to the McCafferys claiming: 'Dana passed away for different reasons than you claim' (ibid.). SAVN was formed in late 2009 in a direct response to the AVN's treatment of the McCafferys and had some links to Australian Skeptics Inc. (ASI).

ASI is an organisation for 'like-minded people to gather and become active […]. They address the whole range of quackery, which is everything from homeopaths through to psychics and water diviners' (McLeod, interview with author, 2017). These pseudoscience sceptics investigate and challenge paranormal claims, making the argument that their movement was necessary because scientists have not taken responsibility for countering anti-science views (Loxton n.d.). A number of those on the ASI committee have been involved with SAVN, although it was independently formed and has adopted a broad constituency, with over 15,000 followers on Facebook as of 2024 (it appears to have dropped from over 64,000 followers in 2019). Rachael Dunlop, a SAVN and ASI member, is a senior researcher at Brain Chemistry Labs (Institute for Ethnomedicine, Wyoming, United States). Known as 'Dr Rachie' in her pseudoscience sceptic work, she has published articles in the mainstream media supporting vaccination (Dunlop 2013a,b).

Other members of SAVN have less connection to pseudoscience sceptics. SAVN is unusual in its wide and varied membership. For example, philosopher Patrick Stokes recounts: 'I started interacting with the SAVN Facebook page [...] and I wrote a piece for The Conversation. That became quite popular and, through it, I ended up being sort of involved more and more within the administration of SAVN, and then some of its activism campaigns' (Stokes, interview with author, 2017). Ken McLeod became involved following a career in air traffic control as a senior manager and later whistleblower: 'I was used to whistleblowing in political activism. I stimulated a couple of Senate enquiries and it just seemed a natural drift [...] my baby sister had polio. I was very young and so I'd seen what happens up close' (McLeod, interview with author, 2017).

Thus, McLeod had both a personal connection to the trauma of disease seen as being vaccine-preventable and ample experience in pushing for policy change. He felt that outlining a social ill to the public was not enough, and they 'needed to do something' to stand out from other pro-vaccine groups that focus on education and 'just giving the facts' (McLeod, interview with author, 2017). Facebook offered an initial forum to counter the AVN, followed by other online strategies, including a 'Google bomb' (manipulating AVN Google searches to result in pro-vaccine websites, by giving those sites a high search rank). Dunlop calls it 'being proactive rather than reactive', to 'prevent the passage of info from professional anti-vaccinationists to the public' by 'those who profit from promulgating antivaccine ideas' (Dunlop, email correspondence, 2017). Thus, SAVN aimed to 'drive these people out of business' (Dunlop, interview with author, 2017). They directly oppose vaccine-critics, undermining them financially, legally, and as a credible knowledge source.

SAVN is keen to point out that this aim is justified because the AVN is not some typical non-profit parent group but a for-profit endeavour seeking to make money from reading materials, talks, and donations. SAVN has not only been active online but also attempted to cut off AVN platforms and income sources by contacting the AVN's venue hosts and sponsors, by pursuing legal action, and through policy means. Following a complaint, the Australian Office of Fair Trading deemed the name 'Australian Vaccination Network' as misleading and a detriment to the community, causing AVN to rename itself the Australian Vaccination-Skeptics Network. The McCafferys and also SAVN filed a formal complaint to the Health Care Complaints Commission (HCCC) for the AVN's spreading of misinformation: 'The HCCC found against the AVN and issued a public warning about the group in July 2010. The AVN lost their charitable status as a result, but won it back after a NSW Supreme Court challenge ruled the HCCC did not have the jurisdiction' (Health Care Complaints Commission 2014). The government quickly amended the relevant legislation, and the public warning was reissued to cancel AVN's charity licence from the Office of Liquor, Gaming and Racing.

These outcomes indicate a supportive pro-vaccine environment in Australia. Rachel Heap, a specialist in intensive care medicine who is part of the pro-vaccine group NRVS, believes that news outlets have become less likely to adopt a 'false balance', raising the profile of minority views by allocating the same time and attention to both sides of the vaccine debate (interview with author, 2017). Australian politicians have also become more comfortable speaking in support of vaccination, and two policies – 'No jab, no pay', removing child benefit payments (and non-medical exemptions), and 'No jab, no play', restricting state day care – aim to curb falling vaccination rates (Beard, Leask, and McIntyre 2017). However, grassroots activists have been less directly involved in these policy changes, which have origins in their current form from media campaigns by Australian newspaper the *Daily Telegraph* as well as the *Sunday Edition* (Hansen 2013b).

Perhaps indicating journalistic policy origins, many local health officials I spoke with viewed these policies as populist and not particularly helpful in the long term, further polarising the vaccination debate and hindering discussion between both sides (also see Leask and Danchin 2017). Thus, there are other considerations that result from instituting coercive policy. Indeed, the deviant 'problem publics' are the vaccine critics, and this is why they receive the most attention in how allegedly false beliefs can persist while being in the minority. Unlike the vaccine critics, pro-vaccine activists are not problematic but seen to be the 'rational actors' and are hence overlooked. However, they can offer an insight into unfolding vaccination debates and reactions to anti-vaccine ideas.[14]

Making sense of pro-vaccine activism

These case studies can be distinguished from other examples of vaccination views and behaviours in asking two questions: What are the reasons for, impacts sought by, and implications of pro-vaccine citizen activism? And what wider political, social, and moral arguments are conveyed? To address these questions, I consider the means, message, and motivation of pro-vaccine activism and importance of taking a country-level view. First, the means of pro-vaccine activism in these cases have consisted of a significant amount of online activity alongside offline mobilisation. In the United States, certain vaccinations are mandatory for enrolment in public schools and day-care, with varying exemptions applied at the state level, whereas in Australia this has historically not been the case, although it is beginning with day-care. The legal entrenchment of vaccination in the

14 I refer to such an account as a 'symmetrical' analysis in the sense popularised by David Bloor (1991). He argued that, when analysing a scientific controversy, it is important for each side of a competing knowledge claim to be treated equally through social analysis and not as being either true or false. Inspired by this idea of symmetry, I analyse a side of a debate not usually observed because it is perceived as being on the 'right' side of scientific understanding. Such an approach is connected to Bloorian symmetry by not assuming pro-vaccine views and behaviours are the correct knowledge, thus not needing enquiry.

United States means the battle lines differ from those in Australia, where activism can be very broad in influencing state policy. The American vaccine debate mostly plays out heightened discussions of exemptions to vaccination across states. In Australia, by contrast, persuasive routes using media influence are most common; however, increasingly more regulatory routes are being employed, such as withholding welfare payments and state childcare provision to those who do not vaccinate, and not allowing for any non-medical exemption. Against this backdrop, both of the activist groups are coercive in character, yet focus on different targets – SAVN being coercive in their activities towards the AVN through active countering and trying to shut them down, and Vaccinate California wanting to enact more coercive policies by tightening the vaccine exemption law.

Second, the message that each group has attempted to convey differs substantially and points towards sources of cross-country differences. Framing a particular message is used to both galvanise collective action (Benford 1993) and set boundaries for that action (Silver 1997). The message of Vaccinate California falls under an education and safety frame. The 'safe school' argument overrides the right for choice in public spaces and derives from a collective idea of parenting and care for children (at least in a minimal sense of not causing harm to other children). Such a parenting view, firstly, is connected to values upholding science, evidence, and state authority; and, secondly, it means that activists can disengage with directly opposing viewpoints and avoid explicitly addressing competing knowledge claims. Direct oppositional activity seen in Australia has been less prevalent in the United States.

Likewise, while Vaccinate California played a crucial role as the parental mandate to pass SB 277, there are limits to this type of activism, as no equivalent lobby exists nationally. I make this point to highlight not only the system of vaccination policy within American states but also the connection of political culture to opportunity structures for resource mobilisation (see Goodwin et al. 2003). In the United States, the policy environment is not amenable to a group directly countering vaccine critics, like in Australia. As Dunlop saw it, a group like SAVN could only really be successful in Australia and would not find a foothold in the United States (interview with author, 2017). It is not only that the scale of organisation and resources needs to be greater to make rhetorical arguments; such argumentation would also need to stand up against freedom of speech. This is constitutionally enshrined and individual choice often elevated as an ideal above 'big government' in ways that create difficulties for pursuing notions of the common good. Indeed, sociologist Jennifer Reich frankly concludes in her 2016 book that Americans do not see community support benefiting them, rendering collective responsibilities irrelevant, although, as I have shown, a concept of collective parenting concerning public spaces does exist. SAVN's message, by contrast, falls under a pro-science frame. Their stance is scientific, expert, and evidence-based, and the opposition is 'loony', crank, and pseudoscientific. It is a broad-based constituency that can move away from the issue of parental autonomy over health decisions and the safety of risk judgements made. Upholding pro-science values is a bigger focus than a reiteration of the importance of vaccination itself, which is taken as given. The emotional intensity of grieving parents being under attack gives added moral legitimacy to the cause.

The implications of these differing styles of activist citizen approaches in support of vaccination are shown in SAVN's moral indignation as combative, with little discussion or attempt at understanding in-between. Such a position, according to two Australian academics, is detrimental to the long-term public trust in vaccination as questions and concerns are not allowed to surface. Public health academic Julie Leask is concerned about inhibiting constructive debate: 'If we have an attitude of shutting down criticism, then we may have situations when we don't listen when we really need to' (quoted in Bramwell 2014). Sociologist Brian Martin, meanwhile, is critical of methods used by SAVN to silence free speech and discredit individuals through 'verbal abuse, harassment (especially via numerous complaints) and censorship' (2016, p. 27). Even if SAVN does fit this description, and although they have met some pushback, they are still able to be active in Australia. Direct government backing of pro-vaccine groups is generally strong, albeit at arm's length, with some uncertainty over involvement with the activities of groups acting outside of conventional institutional channels. Governments prefer publics to reach broad social consensus on controversial topics (Irwin 2006). Australia, at present, is seeing vaccine promotion crossing major party lines, with a pro-vaccine media able to influence public policy and political rhetoric.

Third, who is motivated to pursue these messages and why? The characteristics of activists not only shape the type of campaign pursued but also reveal their understanding of what it means to be pro-vaccine in their reasoning and objectives. Vaccinate California mainly identify as parents – not unexpected for an issue that typically concerns parents, especially mothers, who often take greater responsibility for their children's health (Ranji and Salganicoff 2014) – whereas SAVN mainly see themselves as science supporters. The reason behind why these pro-science and anti-pseudoscience types of activists have appeared in Australia compared with the United States appears to be related to what pre-existing groups were already in place (e.g. through the ASI) and whether they were able to quickly reorganise to fill a gap for a pro-vaccine entity.

Furthermore, what has motivated these pro-vaccine activist groups to have an impact now? Two reasons present themselves: one, the threat of illness and death from what are thought to be vaccine-preventable diseases; and two, a perceived need to counter vaccine-critical views. Just as vaccine-critical groups mobilise on the basis of perceived harm to children, so do pro-vaccine activists mobilise against perceived harm caused by those who do not vaccinate, rather than in support of the vaccine per se. The trigger for both activist groups was child mortality or threat thereof, connected to low vaccination rates. This remains a motivating factor for supporters of vaccination to step out of the silent majority and become activists. A need to counter vaccine critics is another motivating factor – whether in the treatment of grieving parents or in their dominance in a community outbreak. The fact that many SAVN supporters are similarly supportive of other pro-science issues and countering pseudoscience claims demonstrates that countering vaccine critics is also an act of addressing and penalising views deemed unacceptable in society.

Active support for vaccination through pro-vaccine activism relies on high-profile events as triggers, as well as the provocation of fundamental beliefs concerning, on the one hand, the value of science, evidence, and the state; and, on the other, a collective view of child-rearing or care for children. When not given enough reason to act, the pro-vaccine contingent of civil society remains inactive, typically reactivating in response to media triggers and perception of a larger population affected by vaccine-preventable diseases. However, it is also the long-term accumulation of anti-vaccine views that are profiled in public discourses and through media representation that eventually becomes unacceptable to mainstream publics.

Nevertheless, overall outcomes sought by the pro-vaccine activist groups are similar in that they both push policy and societal change towards more coercive measures to support vaccination. Previous activism or advocacy in civil society has been, on the whole, more information- and education-based. As Attwell and Smith (2017) argue, coercion may be problematic if hard-line policies create tiers of citizenship where vaccine decisions become a marker of identity. The concern is that views critical or wary of vaccination are neglected and their proponents viewed as less worthy citizens. This disregard threatens the relationship of trust between parents and the state, with the potential for a larger backlash in the future.

Overall, pro-vaccine activism has been an unproblematised aspect of the vaccination debate but such activist groups and activities are likely to become more prominent in reaction to the greater perceived threat to mainstream views.[15] The 'counter' nature of this type of activism reinforces how mainstream views are sidelined but also how public health goals are subject to differing interests and structural determinants from a wider political economy of health. How political and economic circumstance impacts vaccination is a wide-ranging question. Societal interaction with vaccination is greatly affected by these structural factors. The next section addresses the earlier stages in vaccine development process, within the context of how vaccines for some diseases have not received the attention that is needed in global health policy.

15 The 'March for Science', for instance, began in 2017 organising rallies/marches worldwide to celebrate science in the face of funding cutbacks and downgraded policy importance. Another parallel of counter-activism within polarised debates seeking government and public support are pro-choice groups getting 'public space protection orders' to prevent harassment by anti-abortion protesters outside clinics in the United Kingdom (BBC News 2018).

Typhoid – an overdue vaccine

This example examines how policy neglect has meant that vaccines have not improved for some diseases. I focus on typhoid fever, first as a neglected disease by addressing why a vaccine had not been developed and second, the role of advocacy on the part of trial participants and international organisations to bring attention to an overdue vaccine. The potential of trial participants to act as vaccine advocates has been overlooked, especially in conjunction with the advocacy work of powerful philanthropic donors who have the capacity to raise health topics up policy agendas. Typhoid fever is a disease that has benefited from increased policy attention. Caused by the bacterium *Salmonella enterica* serovar Typhi, or *S.* Typhi, typhoid infects people through contaminated water and food, causing a range of symptoms such as fever, abdominal problems, and a rose-coloured rash, eventually killing up to one in five of its victims, if left untreated (Kenneth et al. 1993). According to 2019 WHO global figures, each year typhoid affects 9 million people and causes 110,000 deaths (WHO n.d.). While it is a long-afflicting disease of humankind, typhoid persists in many places of poverty where public infrastructure is lacking, but the difficulty in control has been both for technological and sociopolitical reasons.

Technologically, control of typhoid transmission via water and contaminated food is complicated because the bacterium can also be excreted by outwardly healthy people who show no clinical symptoms of typhoid infection. Although these asymptomatic or 'healthy' carriers have no symptoms, they can still excrete *S.* Typhi through their faeces for years after the initial infection. The concept of healthy carriers was advanced by the German bacteriologist Robert Koch in 1902 (Gradmann 2010) and dampened early hopes for typhoid elimination because asymptomatic carriers could put others at risk. They presented a problem for public health authorities who initially thought water, sanitation, and hygiene (WASH) measures would be sufficient. Most typhoid carriers were allowed to remain in their communities if they agreed to follow precautionary measures, such as abstaining from working in food preparation and waterworks, but some were forcibly detained and isolated. Irish immigrant Mary Mallon, who became known as 'Typhoid Mary' (Image 3.10) after repeatedly infecting people through her work as a cook, remains the most publicised case of an asymptomatic typhoid carrier having to be detained (Leavitt 1996). Mallon was depicted sensationally in the press and confined for most of her life on North Brother Island, in New York City's East River (Image 3.11).

Typhoid did continue to decline in high-income countries due to WASH measures and surveillance, including the monitoring of healthy carriers. As time went on, the treatment of carriers rarely made headlines, although unfortunate cases – like the detainment of female carriers deemed mentally incapable of upholding sanitary standards in the Long Grove Asylum in Epsom between 1907 and 1992 – have only more recently come to light (BBC News 1990). By the end of World War II, Europe and North America were combating typhoid with functioning sanitation systems, chlorination, national surveillance of typhoid outbreaks and carriers by public health authorities, vaccines, and effective antibiotics, for example, chloromycetin in 1948 and ampicillin in 1961 (Kalra et al. 2003). Antibiotics also offered a solution to treat carriers who had previously had to rely on 'heroic interventions' such as quarantine and gall bladder removals.

Vaccines for typhoid on a truly global scale, meanwhile, have been more limited. As other interventions had worked well, typhoid vaccines were, until very recently, primarily used for protecting the military and foreign travellers and to limit acute outbreaks in high-income countries (Kirchhelle and Vanderslott 2019a). Those vaccines had been developed to protect populations in areas without sanitary infrastructure, proving particularly useful by World War I, when all major powers used improved typhoid vaccines to protect troops and travellers (Gradmann, Harrison, and Rasmussen 2019). The first live attenuated oral vaccine Ty21a was licensed in Europe in 1983 and in the United States in 1989, followed by a subunit 'Vi capsular polysaccharide' vaccine (ViCPS) licensed in the United States in 1994 and an inactivated Hepatitis A–Typhoid combination vaccine licensed for many countries in 2007 (Freedman, Virk, and Jong 2008) (Images 3.12 and 3.13).

Wealthier countries did not need a typhoid vaccine for mass use. By the early 1900s, many of the cities in high-income countries were investing

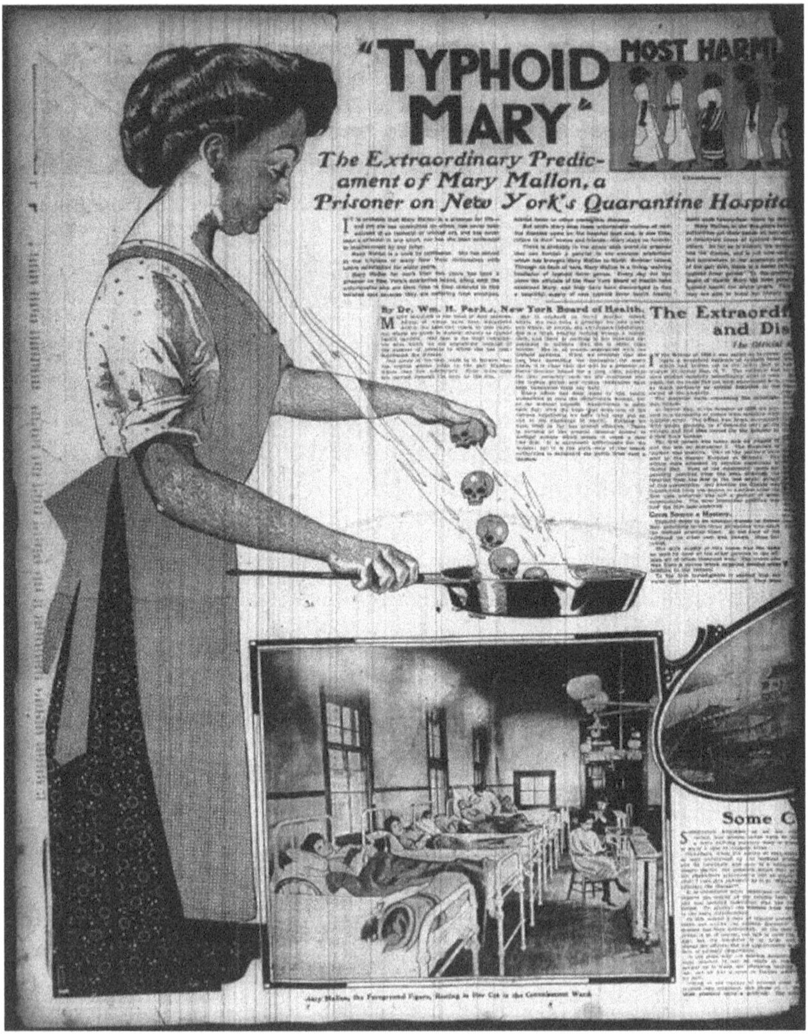

"TYPHOID MARY"

MOST HARM

The Extraordinary Predicament of Mary Mallon, a Prisoner on New York's Quarantine Hospita

By Dr. Wm. H. Park, New York Board of Health.

The Extraordi

and Dis

Some C

Image 3.10 'Typhoid Mary' in the press.

General Research Division, New York Public Library. 'Typhoid Mary', the New York Public Library Digital Collections. 1909-06-20. <https://digitalcollections.nypl.org/items/85674452-ba9e-6934-e040-e00a1 80606cf>

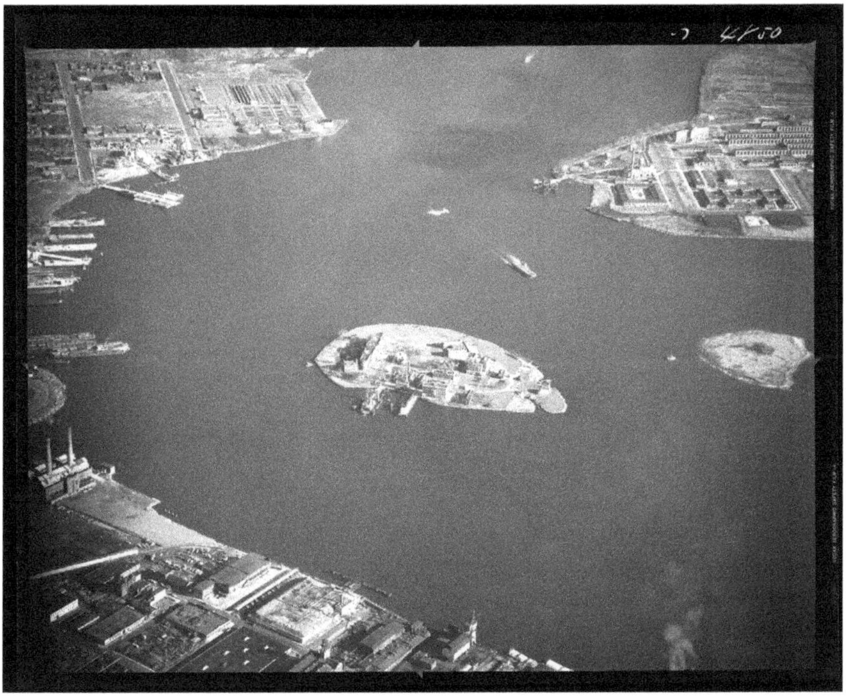

Image 3.11 Aerial image of North Brother Island.

New York State Archives, aerial photographic prints and negatives of New York State sites, 1941–57, B1598–99. Box 8, no. 52.

in water and sanitary infrastructures, and despite some hit-and-miss interventions, there is a clear correlation between rising expenditure on the provision of safe water services (including treating the water supply with chlorine) and declining mortality from waterborne diseases (Vanderslott et al. 2019). Populations in poverty without access to clean water and sanitation are most impacted by typhoid. Other reasons may also have contributed to mass immunisation being limited. The typhoid vaccines developed were not suitable for young children, and the perception that typhoid fever is only a childhood disease may have reduced the appetite for large-scale, all-ages vaccination efforts (Garrett et al. 2022).

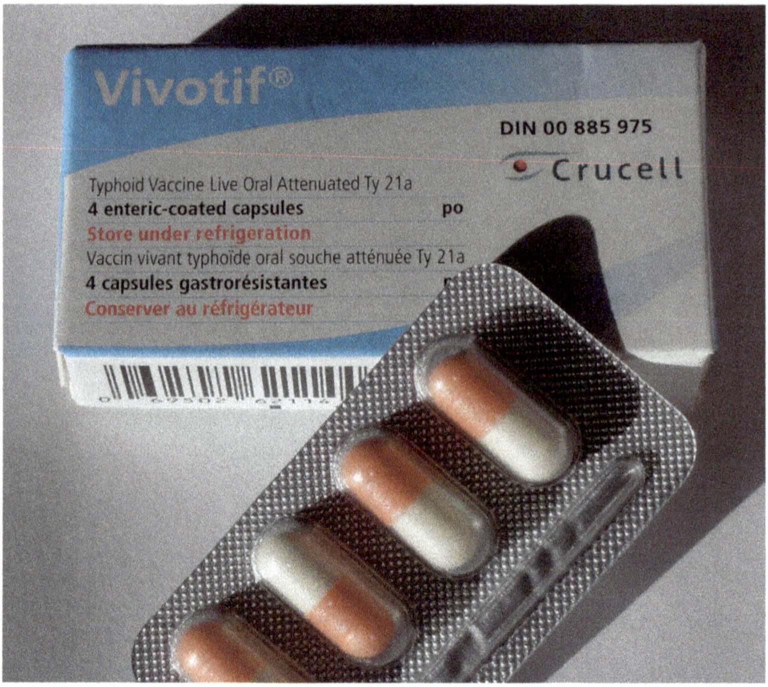

Image 3.12 Vivotif, a live attenuated bacterial vaccine against typhoid.

Wikimedia Commons/CC-BY-SA-3.0.

It is clear then that steps towards typhoid elimination have depended on both long-standing and new technologies to prevent, diagnose, and treat the disease. WASH, for example, is a long-used preventative intervention, but investment in poorer countries has not been enough to eliminate typhoid. Typhoid had almost vanished from high-income countries, mainly through the use of such long-standing technologies but has remained endemic in other parts of the world. This infectious divide has been reinforced by a relative neglect of international campaigns to tackle typhoid, such as the sustained large-scale investment in the supply of safe drinking water, safe sewage disposal, and basic healthcare services. Investment has often remained ad hoc, uncoordinated, and insufficient, with many wealthier countries focusing on their own protection by prioritising vaccines

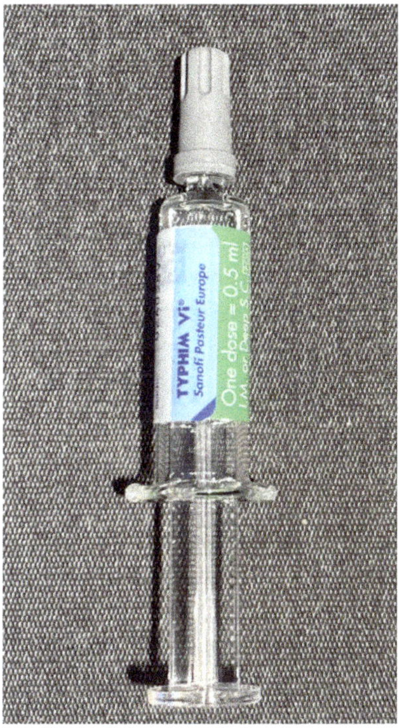

Image 3.13 TYPHIM Vi solution for injection.

for specific populations. Along with antibiotics and surveillance-based biosecurity regimes, efforts have concentrated on stopping typhoid from crossing back into high-income countries via travellers and migrants. Such an inward-looking nature of Western disease elimination and eradication campaigns over the past century has meant typhoid control stopped at high-income borders, to become a neglected disease in other, poorer countries (Kirchhelle and Vanderslott 2019b).

While investment in long-term solutions has been lacking, the over-reliance on relatively cheap antibiotics to control typhoid has resulted in increasingly antibiotic-resistant strains. As Kirchhelle et al. (2020) argue, industry marketing and targeted campaigning have encouraged inappropriate antibiotic usage. In places lacking in healthcare systems and social security, people also use antibiotics because they have no alternative that they can afford. New extensively drug-resistant (XDR) variants of typhoid fever that are resistant to at least five antibiotic classes have spread across borders. Such drug resistance means that it is becoming increasingly difficult to treat typhoid, and total pan-resistance of typhoid to locally available oral drugs may be only one mutation away (Kirchhelle, Dyson, and Dougan 2019). In addition, international trade and travel make it inevitable that a regional rise of antibiotic resistance will have global knock-on effects. This problem is further compounded by under-reporting and international surveillance gaps, meaning that drug-resistant typhoid may be even more widespread than previously thought. Travel-related cases have been reported in many countries, including the United Kingdom, Germany, Australia, Canada, and the United States (ibid.). Many travellers had become infected visiting Pakistan, where there has been a large-scale outbreak of XDR typhoid, with at least 5,274 cases in the Sindh Province since 2016 (Image 3.14). A warning signal had already been sent in the form of a large outbreak in Kashmir in 1988, resistant to all three first-line antibiotics, followed by similar outbreaks in Shanghai, Pakistan, and the Mekong Delta (ibid.). The Pakistani XDR strain is now showing resistance to all commonly available antibiotics except azithromycin and carbapenems (Butt et al. 2022).

Alarmingly, in November 2019, the first case of a person in the United States with no history of international travel was confirmed, and by 2021 a total of nine cases of XDR-typhoid not linked to travel had been identified (Hughes et al. 2021). These non-travel-related, antibiotic-resistant cases are likely to increase. Many would have thought a disease like typhoid would no longer pose a threat to higher-income countries, as sanitary improvements, effective vaccines, and antibiotics had previously eliminated endemic typhoid. Nevertheless, expanded vaccine use offers a route to reduce dependence on antibiotics, in addition to continued commitment to WASH and other interventions. In comparison to antibiotic resistance, there is less time for a pathogen to evolve as the body is already prepared to fight off an infection and is why vaccine resistance has tended to be less of a worry (Kennedy and Read 2018). Vaccines thus present opportunities for less reliance on antibiotics, with the ultimate goal of decreasing both

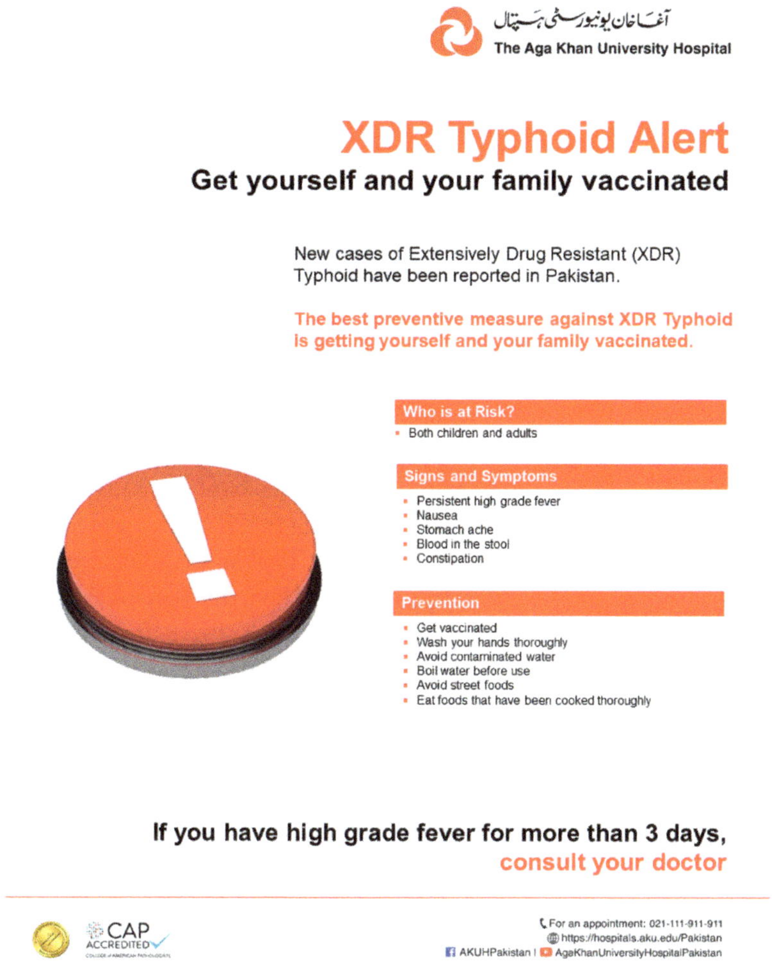
آغا خان یونیورسٹی ہسپتال
The Aga Khan University Hospital
XDR Typhoid Alert
Get yourself and your family vaccinated
New cases of Extensively Drug Resistant (XDR) Typhoid have been reported in Pakistan.
The best preventive measure against XDR Typhoid is getting yourself and your family vaccinated.
Who is at Risk?
Both children and adults
Signs and Symptoms
Persistent high grade fever
Nausea
Stomach ache
Blood in the stool
Constipation
Prevention
Get vaccinated
Wash your hands thoroughly
Avoid contaminated water
Boil water before use
Avoid street foods
Eat foods that have been cooked thoroughly
If you have high grade fever for more than 3 days,
consult your doctor
CAP ACCREDITED
For an appointment: 021-111-911-911
https://hospitals.aku.edu/Pakistan
AKUHPakistan | AgaKhanUniversityHospitalPakistan

Image 3.14 Extensively drug-resistant (XDR) typhoid alert.

The Aga Khan University Hospital. <https://hospitals.aku.edu/pakistan/AboutUs/News/Pages/XDR-Typhoid-Alert.aspx>

the incidence of infections and the number of antibiotics needed for any given treatment (Lipsitch and Siber 2016).

A renewed investment in typhoid vaccines came from the 1990s onwards, and the United States was investigating a new live oral typhoid vaccine in the early 2000s, driven by pharmaceutical companies in middle-income countries, supported by trial participants in high-income countries. Bharat Biotech, an Indian company, began testing typhoid vaccines around 2010. It was a reversal of long-standing global power dynamics, as Indian biotech companies are now at the forefront of new vaccines for typhoid. Bharat Biotech's Typbar typhoid conjugate vaccine (TCV) was the first to gain international approval (after Bio-Med's PedaTyph vaccine had been licensed only in India by 2011) (Sahastrabuddhe and Saluja 2019). The Typbar TCV phase III trial took place between 2011 and 2012 (Mohan et al. 2015), and on participants in Oxford, United Kingdom in 2017, followed by further large-scale trials in Nepal and India (Image 3.15). There are many other TCVs in development, including PedaTyph, as well as collaborations with big pharma companies. When Typbar TCV received WHO prequalification in 2018, it was supported by Gavi, the Vaccine Alliance for introduction into other countries. The fact that a single-dose vaccine was now available for children as young as six months old was seen as a major breakthrough in the control of typhoid, and had shown to induce around 82 per cent protection (Meiring et al. 2019). The mass rollout of the vaccine to over 10 million schoolchildren in Pakistan began in late 2019, in an attempt to control the Sindh Province XDR outbreak (Qamar et al. 2020). As of 2024, there are three WHO-prequalified TCVs that are effective for all age groups, require only one shot, and do not cause large-scale side effects. Therefore, the development of a 'next-generation' of vaccines coming from a middle-income country has opened up new possibilities for typhoid control.

Next, I introduce the role of trial participants in advocacy, and specifically their participation in 'human challenge studies' (also known as a controlled human infection models or challenge trials), where a person is intentionally infected with a pathogen in a controlled environment to

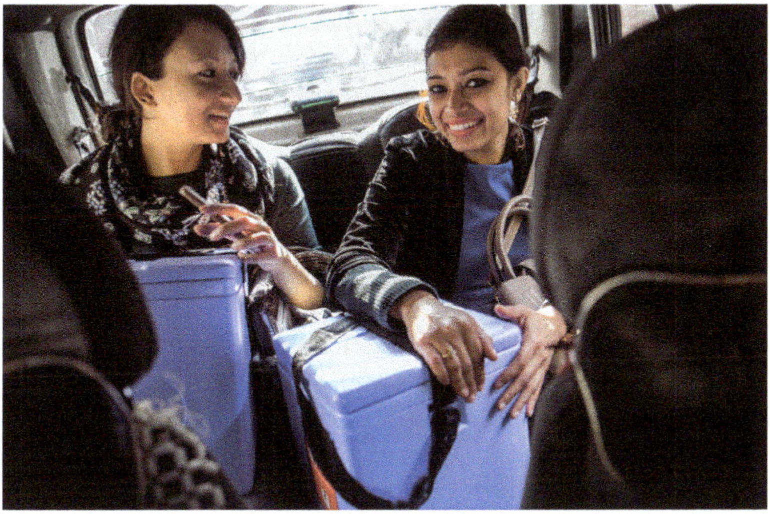

Image 3.15 Bringing typhoid vaccines to Nepalese trial sites.
Photographed by Samantha Reinders.

test a vaccine or learn more about a disease.[16] The role of trial participants for vaccine communication will also be discussed in the following section on COVID-19 vaccines. This introduction to participants emphasises the importance of people who provide their bodies for the testing of vaccines. The University of Oxford typhoid trial helped to support decisions about policy and licensing of a new vaccine that was being implemented in places where the disease posed a substantial threat.

Vaccine trials usually involve rolling out a new vaccine to what amounts to thousands of people (in later stages of the trial or 'phase III') and relying on uncontrolled natural infections to test their efficacy. A different approach is to vaccinate and then intentionally infect healthy volunteers under careful supervision for so-called challenge studies. This allows researchers to quickly see how well potential vaccines may work in comparatively safe

16 This section draws on work with Claas Kirchhelle (Kirchhelle and Vanderslott 2019b; 2021).

circumstances. However, there are many considerations to address before going ahead. Challenge studies still require confirmation via phase III and beyond to see the benefits of vaccination at a population level and are not sufficient proof of safety alone.

A geographic shift has been occurring with the new typhoid vaccines, as although they were first developed in higher income countries, many are now being created in middle-income countries but tested in higher-income ones. As touched upon earlier, the Indian Typbar-TCV was tested in Oxford in 2017. This challenge study involved over 100 people drinking live typhoid bacteria to test the new vaccine (Image 3.16). Trial participants noted that they were motivated by the idea of helping and progressing science, especially for vaccines. They did, however, note that this was not a purely altruistic activity, and they would not have taken part without the financial compensation (Boxes 3.1 and 3.2).

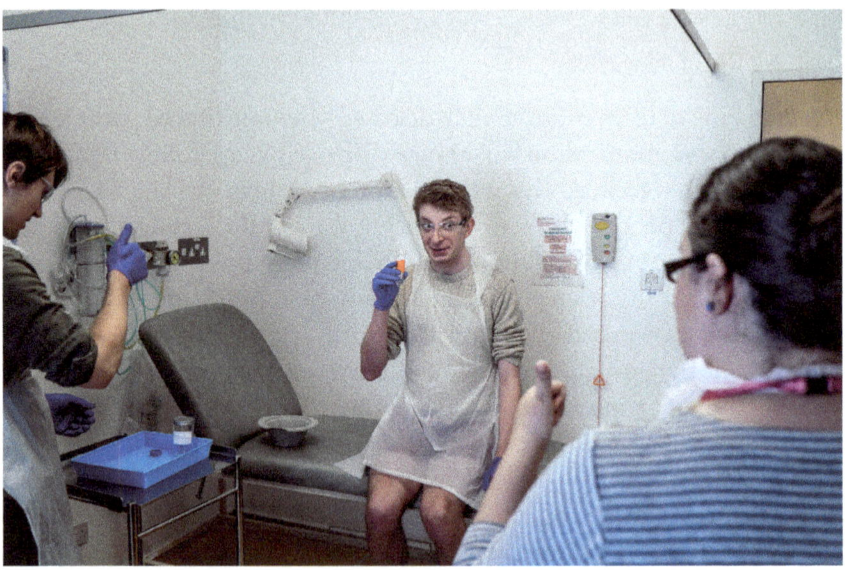

Image 3.16 A volunteer prepares to swallow a vial of live *Salmonella enterica* serovar Typhi.

Photographed by Andrew Testa.

Box 3.1 Quotes about trial participant motivations

Having something like a vaccine trial, where you can get the concrete feeling, that yes, I am actually making a difference with this … So I would absolutely take part in future trials, in fact I actually signed up for my second trial the day that the first trial finished. (Nick, Typhoid Swallowers 2020)

I'm very much interested on a personal level in communicating science and making people understand the importance of science of vaccines, especially in the current anti-vaccine climate and whatever I can do personally, even if it's taking part in a vaccine trial that's my personal contribution to hopefully helping eradicate some diseases … Especially I would recommend women taking part in clinical trials, because the patient or experimental subject cohorts in various clinical trials, women are extremely underrepresented there's different hormone levels, there's different body compositions or all of those aspects really affect the science behind it, so that's definitely worth taking part in trials for. (Daina, Typhoid Swallowers 2020)

Box 3.2 Quotes about trial participant financial compensation

In terms of actually, you know going through the process of catching say typhoid or malaria, you know these very can be really quite unpleasant experiences that having the financial incentive really helps in terms of recruitment for things like that. (Nick, Typhoid Swallowers 2020)

I probably wouldn't have done the trial if it was without any compensation. (Daina, Typhoid Swallowers 2020)

Challenge studies have been conducted for other diseases such as cholera, shigella, influenza, and malaria, with the number of studies increasing over recent decades (Darton et al. 2015). In a historical context, challenge studies are not new to vaccine development. Edward Jenner, the father of modern vaccination, tested a vaccine for smallpox in a similar way in 1796, leading to a vaccine that saved countless lives and paved the way for the eradication of smallpox by 1980. However, Jenner's human challenge experiment certainly was not controlled, and its ethics were questionable from our current vantage point. Jenner originally tested his cowpox vaccine, which provided cross-infection protection against the deadly smallpox virus, on his gardener's son, James Phipps, inoculating him and then exposing him to smallpox (Riedel 2005). Today, such an experiment, even if proven successful and resulting in a new form of vaccination, would likely be questioned ethically. Like other forms of medical experimentation, these infection studies have a mixed history in regard to ethics, and there are also present ongoing ethical challenges even for diseases where treatments are available (thus reducing the risk for participants).

The chequered past of challenge studies stems from a colonial legacy in the nineteenth and twentieth century, where imperial powers trialled new vaccines and treatments on colonial subjects not necessarily through challenge studies, but by actively infecting subjects to conduct 'natural experiments' (Velmet 2020). Vulnerable populations in rich countries were also exploited. It was routine for researchers in the United States to test on prisoners, such as during the 1940s, when 400 prisoners were infected with malaria to test potential treatments (Comfort 2009). In Nazi Germany, doctors conducted infection studies on concentration camp inmates (Roelcke 2004). Even following the 1947 Nuremberg Code (Weindling 2001), which established the principles of informed consent, voluntary participation, and freedom to leave a study, infection studies on prisoners continued in the United States until 1976 (Cohen 2016). Also, the Tuskegee Syphilis Study of African American men (1932–1972)– where 439 men with late-stage syphilis and 185 controls without the disease were watched, but not treated – remains one of the major instances of medical research injustice and unethical practice in living memory (Reverby 2012) (Image 3.17). Its consequences persist to this day, particularly among ethnic

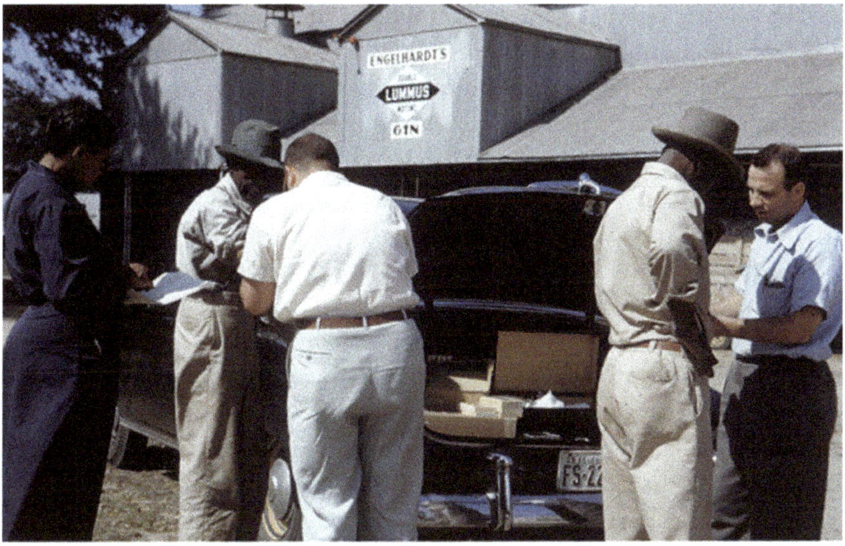

Image 3.17 Participants and researchers in the Tuskegee Syphilis Study.
NAID 956098. 1932–72. The National Archives. <https://catalog.archives.gov/id/956098>

minorities, where mistrust and fear of being misled by health authorities and research persist (Kadambari and Vanderslott 2021).

Issues of exploitation, vulnerability, and financial incentives continue to raise important ethical questions. As Rajan (2017) argues, there are inherent biases in the structures of biomedicine about how health and life are valued amongst different populations, and the governance structures of regulation must therefore be continually reappraised. There are also certain concerns specific to challenge studies, such as the lack of any guarantee that trials will result in successful vaccine rollouts. For example, between 1946 and 1989, Britain's Common Cold Unit infected over 20,000 volunteers with common cold viruses (Greenhough 2012). While the trials improved knowledge of respiratory viruses and led to an anti-influenza compound, they did not result in a proven vaccine (Lambkin-Williams et al. 2018). Furthermore, even when a successful vaccine is produced, trial participants are subject to medical screening to ensure they are healthy before vaccination and infection. This means that for wider populations, there will be varying complicating factors such as age, malnutrition, obesity, or additional infectious and non-infectious diseases (Raymond et al. 2019).

Another problem is the enrolment of trial participants due to limited other options, such as financial and employment opportunities. As sociologist Jill Fisher reports in her book on the social inequalities of clinical drug testing on healthy volunteers in the United States – recruitment is typically from African American and Latin American communities (Fisher 2020). Thus, trial recruitment has been historically an issue affecting a range of marginalised people, from those with no real active choice or knowledge of being enrolled, to those knowingly enrolled but with reduced autonomy, such as conscientious objectors. As Batemen-House points out, for testing on American conscientious objectors during World War II, 'what was voluntary and what was compulsory were intertwined' (2009, p. 594). These experimental subjects, most of whom had chosen 'alternative national service' over military service due to pacifist religious beliefs, were used for testing on typical conflict outbreak diseases affecting both soldiers and civilian refugees, such as typhus (ibid.).

A difficult question today is whether and how to reward participants. The concern is that high financial rewards could unduly influence volunteers to participate in trials due to financial need, and whether low-income countries participants should receive similar payments to those in high-income countries (Raymond et al. 2019). For example, malaria challenge studies have been increasingly conducted in low- or middle-income countries where malaria is endemic (representing a significant public health burden) and there is a dire need for more effective vaccines and therapies. The high burden of malaria disease and deaths and modest efficacy of recently developed malaria vaccines contribute to the perspective of such studies presenting less risk or harm to participants, who would have had prior exposure to the infection (Jao et al. 2020).

A new development for challenge studies has been how they have also become a way to indicate support for the fast development and testing of vaccines. For example, during the COVID-19 pandemic, online campaigns (e.g. <https://1daysooner.org>) demonstrated that volunteers were willing to accelerate COVID-19 vaccine development through the use of challenge studies. In a study by Marsh et al., they found that those who expressed interest in participating in COVID-19 challenge studies 'exhibit consistently altruistic motivations without any special indication of poor risk perception or economic vulnerability' (2022, p. 1). Even while lacking a known cure and proven treatment, volunteers were willing to be infected in pursuit of a vaccine.

However, the ethical goalposts can be subject to shifts when there is political or societal pressure. On an ethical basis, COVID-19 infection studies at the beginning of the pandemic were on the edge of acceptability in requiring knowledge of the appropriate infectious dosage with which to test a vaccine, as usually a 'rescue remedy' is required if participants fall ill, and this was not available at the time. Also, the critical questions in relation to the political economy of where to conduct trials and how to select participants persist. Thus, the development of vaccines against new diseases like COVID-19 will continue to test the ethical limits of existing trial frameworks (Eyal, Lipsitch, and Smith 2020).

Currently, there is no international regulatory framework for challenge studies. In countries such as the United Kingdom, challenge agents are not considered drugs, and studies including no new investigational medicinal product only require local ethics approvals. In other countries, such as the United States, trials are subject to oversight by the Food and Drug Administration (FDA). In low- and middle-income countries such as India, there have been ongoing concerns about the 'offshoring' of clinical trials (Jamrozik and Selgelid 2021). This worry has led to legal restrictions in India, but legalising strictly controlled challenge studies has now been reconsidered (ibid.). It is difficult to say whether this is a self-imposed limitation or whether the worry is justified to avoid predation by pharmaceutical companies wanting quick and easy data, but ultimately phase III and IV will still be necessary.

As COVID-19 and the prospect of future novel pathogens have shown, enormous hopes rest on rapid trials, which means that pressure for challenge studies is growing. In addition to personal hazards for volunteers, there remains a risk that rushed, badly designed, or exploitative studies could undermine wider trust in resultant vaccines and medical research generally. As past experiences such as the 2019 CRISPR-baby scandal show (Cyranoski 2019), weak standards in one place can bring disrepute on an entire community. It is for this reason that the WHO has published criteria (Jamrozik et al. 2021) for the ethical acceptability of COVID-19 challenge studies, and the door is now open for more comprehensive global guidance on challenge studies.[17]

Typhoid philanthropy

While trial participants have shown their support for vaccination, particularly through challenge studies, the actions of philanthropic actors have also driven typhoid vaccine development and adoption. In 2016, the Bill and Melinda Gates Foundation funded the Typhoid Vaccine Acceleration Consortium (TyVAC) as a partnership between university groups[18] and PATH, an international non-profit global health organisation. TyVAC's goal is to reduce the burden of typhoid by accelerating the introduction of new typhoid vaccines into Gavi, the Vaccine Alliance–eligible countries (Jamka et al. 2019). The advocacy campaign 'Take on Typhoid' was established by TyVAC and the Coalition against Typhoid (CaT) as a broad call to action to generate support to reduce the global burden and social impact of typhoid, in collaboration with other organisations working on typhoid. Take on Typhoid has been engaging a diverse group of stakeholders across the typhoid, vaccines, WASH, and child health sectors through conferences, campaigns, and partner publications to distribute materials, blog, and educate people about typhoid and vaccines. The campaign has worked to raise awareness and engagement through advocacy and supporting research into new typhoid vaccines, while also promoting the use of effective vaccines already available and recommended by the WHO. Members have been working with local governments to implement and find sustainable funding mechanisms for typhoid vaccination programmes, as well as to improve typhoid surveillance, especially in parts of Sub-Saharan Africa where the typhoid burden is not well characterised. Christopher Nelson, director of the Coalition

17 The WHO and other organisations have been working on scientific and regulatory considerations for challenge studies since 2014.

18 The Center for Vaccine Development and Global Health at the University of Maryland School of Medicine and the Oxford Vaccine Group at the University of Oxford.

against Typhoid Secretariat at the Sabin Vaccine Institute, described the need for increased funding and advocacy activities in support of typhoid:

> The Coalition against Typhoid was established to fill this need. We are dedicated to making typhoid an international priority and to finding solutions to control typhoid now and not another ten years from now. (Take on Typhoid 2011)

The core campaign was created to direct 'messaging, identifying country champions and important national, regional, and local events to connect with the larger typhoid and WASH communities' (Take on Typhoid 2011). Their resources aim to provide answers to questions using the latest data and evidence, and to inspire advocacy for stronger WASH and vaccine programmes, including country-specific resources to support country introduction. However, the difficulty in effective advocacy is in broad messaging and keeping a balanced agenda. The tendency to prioritise the newly available vaccines continues while there is ongoing neglect and continual challenges of implementing WASH. As Im et al. (2022) have argued, now the focus should be on both WASH and newly available vaccines together for a combined approach, as even modest improvements can reduce typhoid risk.[19] The authors urge the need for assessments in WASH to happen alongside typhoid vaccination, especially when evaluating the new vaccines. In summary, while increased advocacy surrounding an overdue vaccine for a neglected disease is welcome, there is a requirement also for the non-pharmaceutical interventions to remain high on the agenda. However, keeping momentum of public support for ongoing diseases of poverty is difficult and public support can be much more apparent during health emergencies. The heightened sense of urgency for awareness and support by the public has become even more apparent in the midst of a pandemic, as discussed next.

19 An added complication is the difficulty in measuring the impact.

COVID-19 – developing vaccines during outbreaks

When viewing wider structures for public engagement and support for trials, much of the focus by social scientists has been on the political economy, in how neoliberal reforms have made disadvantaged people the objects of experimentation for the pharmaceutical industry and in humanitarian medicine, prompting calls for greater transparency and accountability (Elliott and Abadie 2009; Rajan 2005; Rottenburg 2009; Tam et al. 2015). Social science research on trials has raised important sociological and ethical questions about participation, particularly about the role of financial rewards (Mwale 2020), the racial and gender representation of healthy volunteer involvement (Knepper and McLeod 2018), and reasons for trial participation (Rodríguez-Torres, González-Pérez, and Díaz-Pérez 2021; Detoc et al. 2017, 2019).

However, the role of the trial participant, within the representation of trials and their particular composition, has been brought to the forefront through the COVID-19 pandemic. The development of safe and effective vaccines against severe acute respiratory syndrome coronavirus 2 (SARS-CoV-2) has been heralded by some as the big pandemic success story, especially as development happened much quicker than for previous vaccines and has set standards for vaccines in the future (Almond et al. 2020; Bloom et al. 2021). COVID-19 vaccines were developed in such a short time because they built on existing research that has sought to understand coronaviruses (Vanderslott, Pollard, and Thomas 2020). It was fortunate that SARS-CoV-2 has a similar molecular structure to earlier identified coronaviruses such as SARS-CoV-1, responsible for the SARS outbreak in the early 2000s, and Middle East respiratory syndrome coronavirus (MERS-CoV), for which vaccine development work was underway (Ellenberg 2020). The Oxford-AstraZeneca vaccine, for example, used insights gained from developing a vaccine for MERS-CoV, which was already in early-stage clinical trials. The technologies employed in COVID-19 vaccines thus came of age at the right time, and the pandemic has acted as a proving ground for a novel vaccine platform, as these technologies are new but have been researched over the past decade in other trials.

Furthermore, a collaborative approach overcame some of the usual competitive barriers. The fact that Chinese scientists found and published the SARS-CoV-2 genetic sequence put the initial phase of vaccine development on a front foot (Amodio et al. 2020). A combination of resources, funding, and focus brought on by a global pandemic meant time was not wasted waiting for funds or making the case for research attention (Hanney et al. 2020). The time and effort spent arranging industry partners and organising international testing sites happened much more easily because of this concentration of efforts, which extended also to regulation. The frequency of review by regulators allowed an overlap of stages, and vaccines were manufactured 'at risk', where the quantities needed for each stage and for the anticipated rollout were already produced. Advance purchase agreements and preorders bolstered the funding for the vaccine developers.

Regulatory agencies had also been working very closely with vaccine developers, particularly agencies in the United States, Europe, and Japan, which have historically developed capacity in regulating pharmaceuticals (Fonseca et al. 2021). As vaccines are normally given to healthy people, they are among the most closely evaluated medical products. Even pre-trial, they have to pass ethical review boards to be allowed to begin, and data and safety monitoring boards independently assess the trial throughout (Yao et al. 2013). Regulators are able to set out what requirements of efficacy and safety data they will be expecting for approval. For COVID-19 vaccines, regulators conducted in-time assessments as a 'rolling review', so instead of waiting for data to be sent at one time, they received these data incrementally as they became available. Such rolling reviews are a tool that regulators use to speed up the assessment of a promising medicine or vaccine during a public health emergency, and the process happens before a formal application for authorisation is submitted (Mahase 2021).

In addition, there was no problem in recruiting trial volunteers. People were very willing to take part, and the people the COVID-19 vaccines were tested on were a higher number and a broader range of nationalities than is usual for vaccine testing. The demand for an end to the pandemic ensured high attention to developing vaccines, as shown through the intense public, political, and media interest and pressure. The rapid development of COVID-19 vaccines is therefore emblematic of how public support can be mobilised through trials for the benefit of public health.

Vaccine trials and public support

In considering how vaccines have been developed during outbreaks and their public support, it is also crucial to view vaccine trials in their social context. Vaccine trials have a long history and are now well established as a way to critically test the safety and efficacy of new medical technologies. However, the structural features of a trial mean that the focus is on identifying the ideal test subject and triangulating evidence to determine the potential effectiveness (Dixon and Tameris 2018). These structural features mean that there can be a tension between the logic of protocol, healthcare workers or researchers, participants as objects of experimentation, and the wider public (ibid.). Those interested in trial designs and execution do not always consider competing interests, particularly for the wider public, and often this comes too late when trials fail to sufficiently engage and communicate, and where public support is lacking. However, another important role for publics during outbreaks comes during the trial stage for vaccines, when they can signal their support for vaccination through participation in the trials themselves. This section concentrates on the views of trial participants and the wider public as vaccines were being tested during two outbreaks, beginning with Ebola and then for COVID-19.[20]

Previous outbreaks, notably the 2014–16 Ebola epidemic in West Africa, had demonstrated the important role of vaccine trial participants for the public support of vaccination. Vaccination campaigns required a major effort for community engagement during the epidemic. In treatment trials, participants were recruited from an (often narrow) patient base, whereas those in vaccine trials typically came from a broader community (Vanderslott et al. 2021). It is a feature of vaccination being intended as a mass intervention in health populations that wider public support is often needed, compared to treatment aimed at the unwell.

20 In this chapter, I draw on collaborative research from the 'COVQUAL' project. COVQUAL researched COVID-19 vaccine trial participant views, motivations, and experiences (Vanderslott, Palmer, et al. 2021; Vanderslott, Emary, et al. 2021; Thomas et al. 2023), as well as a social media analysis about public attitudes to the introduction of COVID-19 vaccines (Martin and Vanderslott 2021).

The Ebola vaccine trials in West Africa included elements of communication targeting individuals or specific groupings of potential participants such as healthcare workers. There are many different methods that were deployed for communication, which included a designated hotline, information-sharing meetings, community liaison team, and 'participant trackers'. The STRIVE trial, for example, was a phase III vaccine trial that recruited participants from health workers in Sierra Leone, using a designated hotline and information-sharing meetings for potential participants and the wider health workforce (Callis et al. 2018). This trial compared with a community-based vaccine trial, EBOVAC-Salone, which set up a dedicated community liaison team to work closely alongside trial researchers and social scientists. The main role of the community liaison officers was to manage messaging and communication, conditions for participation, and informed consent, through community and household-level meetings alongside community leaders (Tengbeh et al. 2018). Another vaccine trial, PREVAIL, employed 25 Liberians living in the main town trial area as participant trackers to engage in ongoing conversations about daily experiences of being in the trial and highlighted interpersonal, local, face-to-face communication as a critical strategy. The role of these participant trackers was to collect crucial information to determine the names of participants (when in the communities some residents were only known by nicknames), their locations (using descriptions if there were no street names and relying on family and friends to have knowledge of their whereabouts), and the ability to contact them (e.g. a phone number of a local store) (Browne et al. 2018).[21] These trial examples demonstrate the focus on the participants and communities to enable trial success.

An aspect to consider for communication and wider public support is the heightened role of the vaccine trial participant, as seen during the 2014 Ebola epidemic and continued through to the COVID-19 pandemic. The 'clinical trial' – experiments or observations done for biomedical

21 Browne et al. (2018) saw 'effectiveness' in the high participant retention and the success of strategies such as home visits to avoid overt opposition and dissatisfaction but did not comment on the potential of strategies to be intrusive or coercive.

research – reached a status previously unrivalled during the COVID-19 pandemic, bar perhaps the mass-population-scale trialling of the polio vaccine in the 1950s or the public challenges to experimental medicine seen through the HIV/AIDS crisis beginning in the 1980s. Prior to the COVID-19 pandemic, the vaccine development process was less publicly known. Clinical trials saw thousands of volunteers register globally to test COVID-19 vaccine candidates and adverts cast a wide net for volunteers, with spaces filled quickly (Image 3.18).

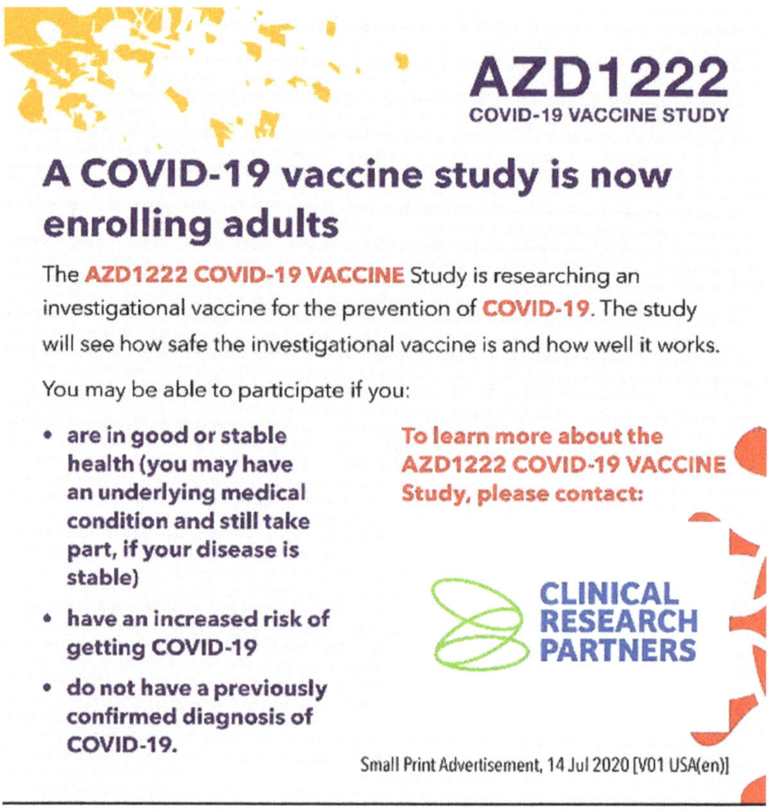

Image 3.18 Advert for Oxford-AstraZeneca COVID-19 vaccine study.

Clinical Research Partners. <https://www.nbc12.com/2021/01/11/astrazenecaoxford-covid-vaccine-study-seeking-minority-participants/>

Such was the attention on trials that governments had to contend with scams attempting to enrol volunteers in order to extract money. The Federal Trade Commission (FTC) in the United States issued guidance for how to differentiate between a real or fake clinical trial (Image 3.19). Despite the interest, clinical trials that are crucial to test new medical technologies and treatments have rarely been uncontentious and without controversy (Kirchhelle and Vanderslott 2021a). Trials involve not only clinical but also ethical concerns, where a balance must be found between the risks and importance of developing safe and validated vaccines. Views on enrolling to take part in research for a vaccine trial reveal individual understandings and negotiations with risk, as well as relations to others via research, with trials also being a way of caring for others and showing altruism. Participants display different configurations of attitudes, beliefs, and emotions (such as hope and trust) in experimentation and testing, as well as negotiating competing cultural values between what Wentzell and Racila (2021) call 'individualizing responsibilization' and 'collective care'. Participants are confronted with individual and collective risks, benefits, and responsibilities to contend with. Such participation in research also forms part of larger

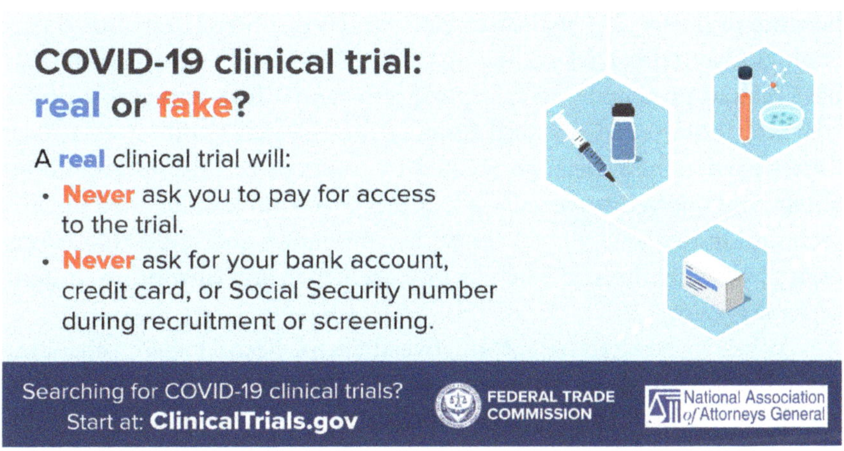

Image 3.19 Consumer alert graphic: COVID-19 clinical trial real or fake?

Federal Trade Commission. (FTC) <https://consumer.ftc.gov/consumer-alerts/2020/10/covid-19-clinical-trial-real-or-fake-learn-how-tell-difference>

processes of different ways or 'everyday strategies' for dealing with uncertainty and risk, including avoidance and intuition (Zinn 2008).

The production of acceptance and acceptability is a central part of trial participation. How participants accept health interventions and their communication about this will be different from the wider public, especially as the people who take part in trials are by default self-selected on the basis of being more highly engaged (e.g. in contributing to medical progress, for whichever reason). Also, while uncertainty is the norm in science, it is not always in line with public expectations and demands, where the use of statistics and calculation of probabilities in the public domain becomes an important component of understanding and management of risk.

Trial participant views

Studies in the past on those who were willing to take part in vaccine trials in non-pandemic contexts (both in reality and hypothetically) have explored motivations and barriers for enrolment (for an overview see Dhalla and Poole 2011). These studies haves identified altruism and the desire for social benefits as key motivators for taking part, as well as personal benefits of protection against disease, which can be related also to psychological and financial well-being (ibid.). Barriers to taking part in trials have related principally to safety concerns and a fear or mistrust of the trial and those organising and funding the research (Mills et al. 2004). Other barriers have been connected to concerns or misunderstandings about study design (especially when this was complex and used unclear technical terms) and worries about discrimination and social risks, along with pragmatic obstacles such as inconvenience and disruption of daily activities (ibid.).

While such research is informative, there has been a focus on analysing participation in vaccine trials for particular diseases such as HIV/AIDs, highlighting the importance of conducting similar studies about participants across vaccine studies and contexts. Trial participation can also provide insight into pro-vaccine views, as I sought to explore, leading the 'COVQUAL' (short for COVID-19 qualitative-focused) project, based at the Oxford Vaccine Group (OVG). We surveyed and conducted semi-structured interviews with participants in a phase I/II vaccine trial of the Oxford-AstraZeneca ChAdOx1-nCOV COVID-19 vaccine (COV001 trial) in Oxford, United Kingdom (Folegatti et al. 2020).[22] Our central interests were in what drove COVID-19 vaccine trial participants to come forward and participate when others did not, their reasons for participation, experience of taking part during the pandemic, and views about vaccination more broadly. The objective of this mixed-methods study completed alongside the COV001 trial was to explore what can be learned from this unusual phase I/II study cohort and the context of their participation, offering wider insights to vaccine trial participation, including for future pandemics.[23]

During the survey and interview period, COVID-19 cases in the United Kingdom had fallen after the first wave but were beginning to rise again. At the time of the interviews, results of the trial had been released showing that the vaccine was safe in humans and immunogenic. Also, prior to their receiving a vaccine as part of the trial, safety and immunogenicity had been demonstrated in animals (Folegatti et al. 2020). Still, it was not known yet whether this vaccine or any other COVID-19 vaccine candidates were efficacious in protecting against COVID-19 disease. The first press release announcing efficacy of any COVID-19 vaccine by Pfizer-BioNTech came out later on 9 November 2020 (Pfizer 2020). Therefore, vaccine efficacy and supply were hypothetical, although Oxford-AstraZeneca had announced a vaccine would be available on a not-for-profit basis. We asked

22 The COV001 trial ChAdOx1 nCoV-19 (NCT04324606) 'first-in-human', multisite clinical trial, which started in April 2020. Between 18 September and 30 October 2020, we recruited from a purposeful sample of 770 healthy volunteers aged 18–55 years enrolled in the COV001 trial who consented to be contacted about further research. We received ethical approval from the University of Oxford Central University Research Ethics Committee (R70147_CUREC). Informed consent was ascertained in writing for the survey and interviews, and verbal consent was obtained for the interview recordings. Interviews took between 45 and 90 minutes to complete.

23 The survey was sent in September 2020, generating 349 responses. We conducted semi-structured interviews with 102 participants led by a team of 11 researchers.

a range of different questions about motivations, views, and experiences of participating in the COVID-19 vaccine trials. Some of the most striking responses were on the topics of 'vaccine nationalism' where participants were asked about how they viewed the supply, and also access to COVID-19 vaccines and taking part in challenge studies.

Participants showed their support for vaccination through a national pride in vaccines developed in the United Kingdom and promotion of the global supply of vaccines according to need. It was a politicised view of national vaccines promoted post-Brexit, as the United Kingdom had left the European Union in 2020, and the government was keen to promote a triumphalist view of a vaccine developed and tested in the country. In interpreting these findings, vaccines are shown to be instruments of power (similar to other pharmaceuticals) in having value not only medically but also as metaphors for facilitating 'social and symbolic processes' (Geest and Whyte 1989). Participants were asked: 'If a vaccine is shown to work, I think people in the country in which it was developed should receive it first' (Vanderslott et al. 2021). Many participants hoped for equitable global access: 'I think it should be given to those who will benefit the most from it, regardless of where in the world they are – any vaccine is a result of cumulative scientific research over decades and contributed to by people all over the globe' (ibid., p. 5). Participants were also asked the open-ended question: 'Should UK citizens receive a vaccine first if it was the country to develop it?' The responses invoked a number of themes, including national pride, a global outlook, prioritisation of vaccine supplies, optimism for a global solution, and politicisation. The balance between national and local was something that participants wrestled with: 'It's a worldwide problem, so I'd be happy if we have a worldwide solution, I don't know how the distribution is going to be done. I guess I would feel a bit bleak if we were at the bottom of the list, but I don't have any problem with sharing it with other nations' (ibid., p. 6).

Many acknowledged that vaccines had taken on a national character, but they viewed the pandemic in an international or global sense. In prioritising vaccines, participants spoke of targeting the most vulnerable and the need for collaboration, but also mentioned that there were reasons for a 'UK-first approach' and a pessimism for a global solution amidst politicisation. While the COVAX initiative[24] was hinted at by some participants, there was not a wide understanding of what that entailed (Image 3.20).

Another question that we asked participants was whether they would agree to participate in a challenge study, which was introduced earlier on in the chapter, and could be thought of as a way of showing high trust and support for vaccines. The question asked was: 'Would you agree to

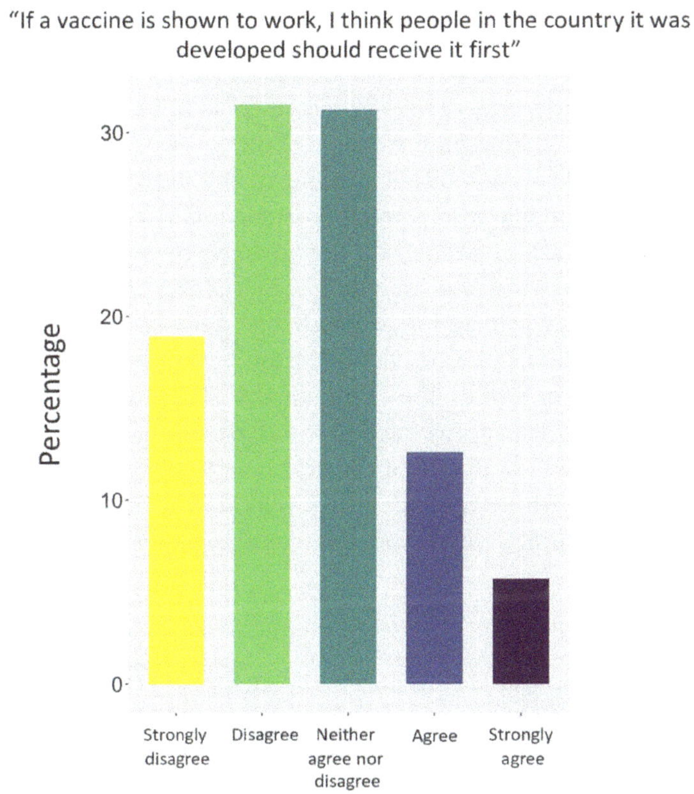

Image 3.20 Survey question on vaccine priority.

Vanderslott et al. (2021).

24 The COVAX initiative by Gavi, the Coalition for Epidemic Preparedness Innovations, and the WHO aimed to support research and development, raised

be intentionally infected after receiving a COVID-19 vaccine to test if it works (this is called a human challenge or controlled human infection model study)?' There was much variation in individual views, although many of the responses focused specifically on perception of risk involved. Some participants viewed the potential public health benefit as sufficient to outweigh potential risk, with the ongoing uncertainty of the pandemic acting as a motivating factor for people to want to participate. This view echoes the principles set out by many ethicists early in the COVID-19 pandemic (Calina et al. 2020) and is in line with the WHO principle to minimise risk and maximise benefit (Jamrozik et al. 2021). These participants appreciated the risk and knew the ethical stakes involved were high in a challenge study, and so they expected trials to be conducted more rigorously and to a high ethical standard (Box 3.3). We found that participant views on risks were multifaceted, mirroring the ongoing discussion among ethicists and scientists. Overall, participants saw the utility in challenge studies and acknowledged these were likely to expedite progress in developing vaccines and understanding the virus causing the pandemic.[25] Some participants saw infection in a challenge study as preferable to community transmission of coronavirus because of its controlled nature of being conducted in a trial. They thought this would maximise benefit, both for personal safety and scientific understanding, at minimal risk. There was a perceived safety of a controlled setting (i.e. in a medical facility) despite the knowledge that there were deaths of people receiving medical care in hospitals. Of those who would consider taking part, some

funding, and negotiated the purchase and distribution of COVID-19 vaccines but did not achieve the cooperation needed.

25 There are limitations to note in representing the views of a small section of the population, who confirmed their commitment to the development of candidate vaccines during the pandemic by enrolling in a phase I/II trial, to be extrapolated to the general population. In addition, as these participants are based in the United Kingdom, their experiences of a COVID-19 vaccine trial may differ from those of individuals in other countries. Finally, this research is based on views gathered prior to the release of data showing any candidate COVID-19 vaccine was effective – this of confirmation may have swayed participants to want to participate.

Box 3.3 Quotes about risk for participation in a challenge study

'I was quite surprised actually because I didn't think there was enough of a reliable treatment for COVID to take that risk, but I imagine they're being very stringent on who they accept in terms of the very, very, very healthy volunteers. I don't think I would do that, but I'm glad that some people do'.

'It's not something that I would imagine that anybody would do lightly in terms of you know, a university or something. You wouldn't do it lightly, and you would have checks and balances, and you would be monitored, all that kind of stuff. Yes, it would be something that I would consider, yes'.

'I think it would do, yes, so how that trial would be run and the support given to the people would definitely be offset, mitigate the risk, and therefore make it more likely that people want to get involved in it'. (COVQUAL project)

said they perceived their risk of developing severe complications as low and did not think a challenge study would cause them harm or disruption. This displays some overconfidence in trial participants as vaccine advocates. They may have a greater 'optimism bias' when a person believes that they are less likely to experience a negative event and do not identify themselves as being at risk (see Fragkaki et al. 2021). Therefore, it is important to consider the type of advocate that a volunteer for a challenge study looks like.[26]

26 The ultimate sign of confidence is perhaps a scientist testing out a new vaccine on themselves, as was depicted in the 2011 film Contagion.

In considering hypothetical participation in a challenge study, participants described an ideal candidate. There were several recurring themes in their responses. Some held the view that a challenge study volunteer must be brave. A minority of individuals interviewed thought that taking part in a challenge study would be an exciting and unusual experience, and they would look forward to sharing this with their loved ones. Others saw their life circumstances as incompatible with participating, despite acknowledging being in good health. For example, being of older age or having dependents were both repeatedly given as reasons why individuals' good health was insufficient. Some expressed the wish for other people to go first, particularly younger people without dependents.

Generally, while vaccine trial participant views were expectedly pro-vaccine, they displayed what it means to support vaccines in a more concrete way. The majority (71 per cent, 246/341) disagreed that it was financial reimbursement that was a personal motivator for taking part (Thomas et al. 2023). Participants were offered between £235 and £625 in financial reimbursement for participation in the study (ibid.), and as Mwale (2017) notes, it is standard practice in the United Kingdom to incentivise participants. The wider public views about the arrival of vaccines also took on a pro-vaccine character, where discourse focused on discussions about hope and the belief for a vaccine to protect against COVID-19. Governments have drawn upon the high hopes for a vaccine to end the pandemic to also stress the need to vaccinate. Although communication by governments and public health authorities to encourage high vaccination rates has attracted critique. The difficulty found in effective communication has persisted, particularly in how to address scientific uncertainty and build trust in health decision making and measures being introduced, and how to implement better public messaging to answer ongoing concerns and worries.

Public views and engagement

When viewing trial participants as vaccine advocates, they will also be situated within a wider discourse about what it means to 'communicate about research' and 'engage the public'. The representation of clinical trials therefore involves a focus on both participant and wider public views and perceptions of trials and the rollout of new vaccines, as well as engagement efforts, situated in historical experiences, health politics and economics. One way of accessing the representation of clinical trials and new vaccine rollouts is through discussion on social media. With my colleague Sam Martin, we analysed social media discussions on X (formerly known as Twitter) about the staged rollout of COVID-19 vaccines across the United Kingdom and United States centred on the arrival for different age groups, with eligibility at different points in time from December 2020 onwards (Martin and Vanderslott 2021). Most of the posts on X were sharing alerts about age group availability, the types of vaccine available, and where they could be accessed. Other discussions were about the safety of different vaccines, including the overall risk of reported vaccine side effects (e.g. for Oxford-AstraZeneca and Pfizer-BioNTech) and how this was still worth the benefit of protection against COVID-19. There were also some prominent examples of pro-vaccine hashtags to emphasise the need to vaccinate, which included: #vaccineswork and #VaccinesSaveslives for general support; #gotvaxxed, #1stjab, and #2ndjab when people received their doses of vaccines; and #Pfizer, #AstraZeneca, or #Moderna to indicate which vaccines people received. There were also discussions of access to vaccines, worry about the number of vaccines available, and whether vaccine passports would be needed to travel and access social events going forward. Therefore, people discuss practical aspects as well as worries and concerns even from a pro-vaccine perspective, and many of the pro-vaccine messages to others were affirming the decision to vaccinate and the importance and trust in vaccines.

Public and community engagement efforts could foster this type of public support. Much of the public engagement activities at present are encouraged by imperatives driven by funders and donors that are aimed at fostering dialogue, appreciation, and mutual understanding between researchers, the research population, and wider public. Some have critiqued this more recent public focus in research, worrying that it can be tokenistic and superficial, and with questions about the value of engagement – not utilising existing support nor engaging in worries and concerns. Anthropologist Sian Aggett (2018) argues for concentrating on the quality and depth of engagement, in the face of logistical and attitudinal obstacles for involving researchers. She makes the point that there is a 'lack of critical conversation regarding the aims and how to achieve them' (p. 307).

Such a two-way perspective for the public understanding of science can be traced to a need to increase research representation and participation, particularly with under-served groups. Still, engagement in health is also situated within wider fields of interest and power, which may or may not permit genuine exchange, community representation, or empowerment. Therefore, developing a critical account of the role that clinical trials and new vaccine rollouts play in navigating and reconciling stakeholder relations for vaccines requires the adoption of the participant and public point of view. Public support of vaccination has played a greater part in the development, testing, and rollout of vaccines than may be initially thought. This chapter has shown the diverse public support for vaccination across four examples: measles and pertussis, meningitis, typhoid fever, and COVID-19, to show the involvement of civil society vaccine promotion for childhood diseases and during outbreaks. An important additional aspect has been the influence of philanthropy, (the mainstream) media, and the political economy. In the next section, I explore how social and online media and community champions are utilised to foster public support, as ways that trial participants and groups can be engaged in communication about vaccination.

CHAPTER 4

Fostering Public Support

This chapter concentrates on how communication about vaccine trials via the media, particularly social media, and communities through 'community champions', is instrumental in fostering public support, from early testing to the vaccine deployment stage.[1] The media plays an important part in representing roles and responsibilities for vaccination, and increasingly the effect of social media is being seen. While community champions have become more prominent in bringing together publics to support vaccination. I discuss the role of the media and social media in portraying vaccine trials and that of community champions in promoting higher public vaccine uptake during rollout campaigns.

Online communication

During 2020 and 2021, the international press was full of articles on vaccine research and developing a vaccine for SARS-CoV-2. A significant focus was on the development of COVID-19 vaccine candidates.[2] In

1 This chapter draws on research on trial participants conducted for the COVQUAL project (Patrick-Smith, et al. 2024) and on community champions (Vanderslott et al. 2024; Kadambari and Vanderslott 2021).

2 This clinical research focus came at the expense of disruption to ongoing and upcoming trials for other diseases across the globe (particularly due to delays to participant enrolment, operational gaps, and complete halts in operations affecting their data integrity and outcomes) (Sathian et al. 2020).

February 2020, when there was a growing public awareness of a potential pandemic, clinical trial efforts and discussions with regulators had already begun.[3] A year later, by February 2021, over 64 candidate vaccines were underway in clinical trials, using a variety of platform technologies (Kyriakidis et al. 2021). The media coverage and public interest in the subsequent COVID-19 vaccine trials has been unprecedented, and public awareness of clinical trials reached an all-time high (Sathian et al. 2020).[4] This intense, and sometimes relentless, media attention and public scrutiny of vaccine trials focused particularly on vaccine safety and efficacy. Such attention also came in the midst of an 'infodemic' – a deluge of information that includes false or misinformation – identified by international organisations, such as the WHO, as an additional threat to infectious disease outbreaks (Buchanan 2020; Zarocostas 2020). The internet and social media can serve as a vehicle to bring information about vaccines to large audiences, which can encourage vaccine hesitancy through false or misleading messages, particularly regarding vaccine safety and side effects (Loomba et al. 2021).

Early calls were made for trials to be transparent so they could be subject to public scrutiny (Mahase 2020). For example, trial protocols were made public, including in some instances the publishing of information sheets and informed consent forms (such as those provided to trial participants by Oxford-AstraZeneca).[5] As Harding et al. argue, this provision of information lacks an account of those taking part in the trials and over-focuses on predefined scientific outcomes, whereas 'the experiences of the participants whose involvement is essential to producing these outcomes are often only heard when a trial ends in glory or disaster' (2021, p. 1). Still, the voice of trial participants has been in high demand, at least in the media, with many appearing on television, radio, and print interviews sharing their experiences. Relatable narratives offer an alternative to

3 In the United States: 'By mid-April, over 70 agents had been registered with the Food and Drug Administration (FDA) for trials of potential treatments, and another 200+ agents were under discussion with the FDA' (Ellenberg 2020, p. 467).

4 Also displayed by the increase in global news mentions in Google search trends, with a particular increase in mentions of 'trial participants'.

5 See <www.covid19vaccinetrial.co.uk/participate-oxford>.

focusing on scientific facts in influencing decision making, and the voice of these participants has been a valuable asset for public health messaging. Therefore, relaying participants' support for research, through societal motivations, and low perceived participation risk is seen as a vital tool in overcoming misinformation and instilling confidence in vaccine development (Wentzell and Racila 2021).

Assessing the roles and responsibilities of different parties is a useful exercise to understand what is involved in communicating about trials. It means seeing where views align and opinions conflict – such a human element and public view of trials is important. The publicity of trials has come into the spotlight, not only through the media and public but also through the high rates of participation and elevated focus on both participants and the teams running trials. It is a publicness that has carried forward a new form of engagement with vaccines. However, a high profile raises a number of questions: What is the nature and scope of mass and social media in covering and representing vaccine trials? How open and transparent are the procedures, participation, and findings? What is the balance between gathering evidence on the one hand, and communication with and involvement of specific public groups on the other? There are also broader issues about the communication of trials that have entered the public sphere in ways that they had not before, which have posed challenges for public confidence and trust in clinical research and vaccine safety. Included here are the speed of vaccine development or progression from preclinical to clinical studies, associated risks and safeguarding, the ethics of animal and human testing, and meeting certain ideals of scientific progress and equity, such as health literacy, evidence-based medicine, and demographic representation (Pepperrell et al. 2021).

The clinical trial has therefore become an important place where evidence generation and scientific developments meet public attitudes and acceptance. However, the change in attention was an unfamiliar working environment for many clinical research teams, as well as the expectation to provide constant up-to-date information to the media, public, and trial participants. The trial participant, the trial team and investigators, the media and social media, and their respective roles and responsibilities have come under the spotlight. All encompass different views and a range of responses about engagement as well as considerations about trials and their involvement. These considerations include the amount of information released to the media, responsibility of using this information, how the representation of the trial both informationally and reputationally is made, and the public confidence or reassurance it espouses.

Stories can be sensationalised, especially in the coverage of trial pauses (when a trial is temporarily suspended), results, and safety. Responsible reporting must be upheld, as it can otherwise put the public perception and integrity of the trials at risk: in how participants and trial teams deal with being under scrutiny, and the balance between publishing every detail of the trial or suggestions of a 'news blackout' until results are ready. The perceptions of participants and their typical interactions with the media and social media affect how they view the trustworthiness of information sources (e.g. from which kinds of news outlets) and use these outlets as tools to inform and educate by sharing accurate information. In addition, the awareness and considerations from media guidance to participants, and if helpful and informative, is important. This guidance includes the perspective on sharing information about the trial on social media and communicating with the mainstream media. A delicate balance must be made between democratising trials and upholding trial integrity.

There are risks in a greater voice for vaccine trial participants and the broader visibility of trials in general. Negative comments about trial participants in popular references in the media have been commonplace, including using descriptions drawing parallels with lab animals who are tested on as 'guinea pigs' (Way 2020). While a trial is ongoing, participants may not be best equipped to cope with a communication role and the attention this may attract. Lynch et al. (2018) note the risks of trial participant social media communication to their safety and for trial integrity. However, a greater visibility of their views and involvement could improve the openness and transparency of vaccine trials, as well as setting an example to reinforce public health messages. There is a possibility of careful management by researchers alongside the clinical study team in obtaining and publicising views. Qualitative-focused studies run in combination with vaccine trials offer an asset for improving vaccine uptake, providing a relatable voice from participants who have an 'insider perspective'. Such public voices could allay concerns and communicate experiences of being vaccinated from a well-informed and relatable collective voice. Potential lies in this group with strong levels of trust in science and a sense of societal responsibility, vaccine trial participants offer a credible voice to support positive messaging around vaccination. Next, I discuss the roles played by the trial participant, the trial team and investigators, the media and social media.

Trial participants

As already introduced in the previous chapter, with colleagues at Oxford Vaccine Group (OVG), we conducted interviews with COVID-19 trial participants in September and October 2020. Interviews were started soon after the trial to test the Oxford-AstraZeneca COVID-19 vaccine was temporarily paused in the United Kingdom on 6 September 2020 following standard processes to review an unexplained illness in a participant (COVID-19 Oxford Vaccine Trial n.d.). The first results from the COV001 vaccine trial were published on 8 December, after the interviews had been completed.

These events were referenced by trial participants, who revealed nuanced views about how they saw their role as ideal test subjects regarding the wider trial itself and representation to those around them and in the media and social media. Overall, they saw themselves as taking an 'altruistic' position in their motivations for wanting to take part (Thomas et al. 2023). The comments made by respondents to our survey suggested that altruistic motivations did not simply refer to the participants' community or nation but also to the wider global community, with participants referring to 'the children', 'the planet', 'anyone', and 'vulnerable people everywhere' (see Boxes 4.1 and 4.2).

Box 4.1 Quotes about participant motivations for participating in the COV001 vaccine trial

'I honestly just wanted to do my bit. I work with young children and I see daily how much this pandemic has affected them and I truly believe that without a vaccine, that won't improve.'

'I just wanted to do my very small bit to help the planet.'

'I lost a family member to COVID shortly before my vaccination and would not wish the experience of losing someone during this pandemic on anyone.'

'My reason for joining the trial was simple: I wanted to contribute in my own way to find a vaccine to defeat a global pandemic. We, the volunteers, are here because we recognise the importance of a vaccine breakthrough and for it to be made freely available for vulnerable people everywhere.' (Thomas et al. 2023, p. 3)

Altruism was also widely understood as spreading positive messaging about the trial. One participant was motivated to share their participation on social media to help with recruitment and raise awareness amongst friends in different cities where the trial was being rolled out out: 'I think I posted at the beginning on Twitter ... when they tried to roll it out across other cities, I shared it because I had a few friends that knew that I'd done it. And they knew that it was happening in their cities' (Patrick-Smith et al. 2024, p. 3). Of those who shared their participation on social media, the vast majority had a positive response and none mentioned receiving any backlash. Many were surprised at the positive reaction, seeing their participation as 'brave' or showing gratitude, and some even found friends or family members shared their participation in the trial on their behalf (it being unclear whether it was done with consent but posts expressed excitement or pride). Participants' perceived role was exposed further in response to seeing others engaging with the media, for example seeing it as a useful way of getting updates on the trial progress. However, others felt that media engagement

Box 4.2 Survey question on motivations for participating in the COV001 vaccine trial

a

	Statement	Strongly disagree % (n)	Disagree % (n)	Neither agree nor disagree % (n)	Agree % (n)	Strongly agree % (n)
Altruistic motivations						
A	I wanted to take action/make a difference/achieve something.	1.7 (6)	1.2 (4)	2.9 (10)	38.1 (133)	56.2 (196)
B	I wanted to help my community/society/country/world.	0.3 (1)	0.6 (2)	1.2 (4)	22.4 (78)	75.6 (264)
C	I wanted to advance the development of the vaccine.	0.30 (1)	0.3 (1)	0.9 (3)	22.4 (78)	76.2 (266)
D	I wanted to contribute to scientific progress	0 (0)	0.6 (2)	2.3 (8)	21.8 (76)	75.4 (263)
E	I wanted to contribute to the improvement of the health of others.	0 (0)	0 (0)	0.6 (2)	23.5 (82)	75.9 (265)
F	I felt a responsibility to take part	0.6 (2)	1.4 (5)	5.7 (20)	38.1 (133)	54.1 (189)
Personal motivations						
G	I wanted a reason to leave the house.	27.8 (97)	22.4 (78)	19.5 (68)	24.4 (85)	27.8 (97)
H	I felt that others would view my participation positively.	5.2 (18)	7.2 (25)	43.0 (150)	33.8 (118)	10.9 (38)
I	I thought that if I caught COVID-19 infection and needed to go to hospital I would have preferential treatment.	75.4 (263)	18.9 (66)	5.2 (18)	0.6 (2)	0 (0)
J	I wanted to tell others about my experience	25.8 (90)	23.8 (83)	26.9 (94)	20.6 (72)	2.9 (10)
K	I wanted to receive financial compensation	47.3 (165)	23.2 (81)	15.5 (54)	12.3 (43)	1.7 (6)
L	I wanted to report my experience to the media	83.4 (291)	14.3 (50)	1.7 (6)	0.3 (1)	0.3 (1)
M	I wanted to receive attention	57.6 (201)	28.4 (99)	10.9 (38)	2.9 (10)	0.3 (1)
N	I was curious about the trial	5.4 (19)	7.2 (25)	14.3 (50)	55.3 (193)	17.7 (62)
O	I wanted to have a new experience	16.1 (56)	18.9 (66)	23.8 (83)	30.7 (107)	10.6 (37)
P	I wanted to access health care/medical attention	54.4 (190)	30.4 (106)	12.6 (44)	2.6 (9)	0 (0)
Q	I was joining a friend or family member who was participating.	58.7 (203)	22.6 (79)	12.0 (42)	5.7 (20)	1.4 (5)
R	I wanted the chance to get the vaccine as it might give me protection against COVID-19.	15.8 (55)	25.5 (89)	27.5 (96)	23.2 (81)	8.2 (28)

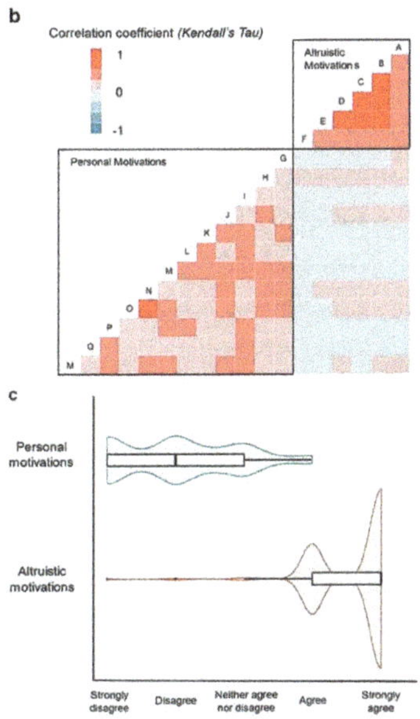

(Thomas et al. 2023)

was not within their remit, as lack of understanding could generate misinformation and in turn damage the trial reputation. An ongoing concern is that participants cannot be effective spokespeople due to lack of knowledge potentially leading to misinformation and to protect the trial privacy some information should not be public. Some thought that the media guidance given by the trial had essentially forbidden contact with the press, and even had an idea that they had signed an agreement not engage with the media, when in fact the media guidance was a recommendation, and not something the trial team asked them to agree to. Additionally, there were some mixed views about those who spoke to the media as either 'attention seeking' or seeking public praise for being altruistic and taking part in the trial: 'I guess like a lot of reasons for people to participate or to tell people is because they want some kind of appreciation for participating ...I think a lot of people do participate because they do think they do something good for society and I guess they want appreciation for it' (Patrick-Smith et al. 2024, p. 3). Participants revealed differing ideas about what their role should be. On the one hand this could be a responsibility to trial privacy not speak to the press nor share their participation on social media, and on the other personal concerns about receiving too much journalistic attention or a backlash from those hesitant about vaccines. However, the mainly positive reflections about trial communication may be particular to the context of large, high-profile trials conducted during a global pandemic. Therefore, while pro-vaccine views might be celebrated especially during times of crisis, this appreciation may not be present in normal times.

Trial team

Participants discussed their views about how the trial team and investigators engaged with the media. Many mentioned specific trial investigators that they had seen and the most frequently mentioned was Professor (now also Dame) Sarah Gilbert. As described in the *Financial Times*, she 'has become the public face of the project – although, like many scientists, she is a reluctant celebrity. She speaks confidently about the project at occasional press teleconferences but interviews are rationed and largely avoid personal matters' (Cookson 2020). The general sense was that the trial team and scientists came across well, instilling confidence and reassurance in the vaccine through their honesty by not being overly optimistic and concentrating on facts, as well as putting across trustworthiness and competency; a view reflected in media accounts (Box 4.3; Image 4.1). Some participants also made more general comments about trust in scientists – but placed the responsibility for improving public trust in science elsewhere, as the role for education or the media.

In Gilbert's book *Vaxxers* (2021) with Professor Catherine Green, the head of the clinical biomanufacturing facility that produced the first batches of the vaccine, she described the high pressure of the media

Box 4.3 Quote by Sky News Science Correspondent about Sarah Gilbert

'Professor Gilbert wasn't weighed down by the responsibility. She was full of optimism, putting the chance of success at 80%. It's rare to find scientists so bullish. They're generally cautious by nature. They speak in caveats. But Professor Gilbert was confident that her vaccine technology could be adapted to meet the new threat. A million doses would be made by September, before the clinical trials were even complete.' (Moore 2020)

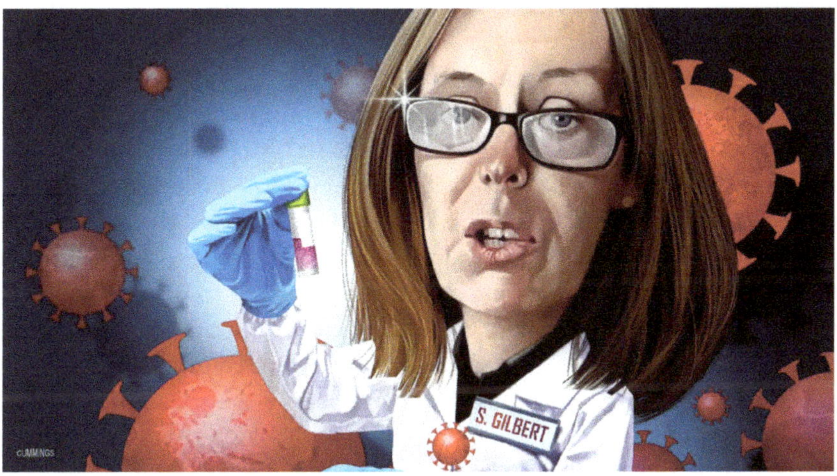

Image 4.1 Cartoon of Sarah Gilbert for the *Financial Times*.

Illustration by Joe Cummings, in Cookson (2020).

and public scrutiny of developing the COVID-19 vaccines: 'Throughout 2020, everyone on the team was stepping up to the task of their life. At the same time because things weren't already hard enough, we were on a steep and sometimes scary learning curve, developing a whole new [media] skill set' (ibid., p. 220). This was repeated by Professor Teresa Lambe, co-developer of the vaccine, who recounted the pressure: 'The search for a vaccine took over my life. I've never worked harder' (Woolston 2020).

A number of participants also remembered some of the interviews that investigators gave to the media, including specific figures mentioned. They recounted that when asked to give an estimate of the likelihood of the Oxford vaccine being successful, Gilbert said that she was 80 per cent sure it would work. This appeared to have stuck in the minds of some participants, with one even thinking that it had been part of the literature given to them by the trial team at screening: 'Think some mistakes were made early on in playing up expectations for the timeline/probability of success of vaccine trials (e.g. talking about this being available millions of doses by Sept 2020, 80% chance of success). don't know how much driven by govt/pharma hype but don't think this was helpful for public understanding' (Patrick-Smith et al. 2024, p. 4). More generally, participants had varying ideas about the level of information that should be released to the media about the trial, including the view that either too little or too much information was reported – for example, reporting on 'non-news' by applying specific significance to trial pauses. The communication about trial pauses was somewhat of a contentious issue as many participants reported that they had received information from the media before being informed by the trial team. For some this was a problem, as they would have liked warning, but most appeared to understand that the media moves so fast that it was often almost impossible for the trial to get the information out to them before it went to press. Participants commented on the media guidance provided by the trial and reported that they had found it helpful.

For some the media should not have much access to the trial details at all, as the 'general public' lacks scientific knowledge to understand the significance or insignificance of day-to-day events. Others felt that the opposite was true, and that regular updates and transparency were important to retain interest and improve public confidence. Some also thought more basic information about how clinical trials work and what a likely timeline for a successful vaccine would look like could serve as an educational service to the public.

Media and social media

The media and social media coverage surrounding COVID-19 vaccine trials was unprecedented. There was a range of responses to questions about the mainstream media and especially its role and responsibilities. Most participants felt the media tended to sensationalise stories, with news being presented as more extraordinary than it actually was – particularly with regards to the trial being paused (or suspended – although more balanced reporting was also found) (Box 4.4). However, some researchers have reported that news sensationalism was low overall, as Mach et al. (2021) found for the United Kingdom, United States, and Canada. Nevertheless, media sensationalism was reported by Scoy et al. (2021) to have caused public anxiety and mistrust in COVID-19 messaging early in the pandemic. Similarly, Dudley et al. (2021) caution that media sensationalism exacerbates even minor flaws in scientific messaging.

Generally, the mainstream media was thought by some participants to have at times reported irresponsibly about the trial, motivated by profit rather than responsible reporting about public health, and so expressed anger and frustration that reputation of the trial was put in jeopardy. Others felt

Box 4.4 COVID-19 vaccine trial headlines

Oxford vaccine trial on hold because of potential safety issue. (Miller and Edwards 2020)

Oxford coronavirus vaccine trial on hold after suspected adverse reaction. (O'Neill 2020)

3 Covid-19 trials have been paused for safety. That's a good thing. (Zimmer 2020)

Covid-19 clinical trial pauses 'show the system is working'. (Hernandez 2020)

they had not seen many examples of irresponsible reporting but added that they avoided certain kind of news outlets for this reason.

The unusual amount of media interest in this particular trial was pointed out by participants, who felt that clinical trials are not usually so prominent and hence the media are not informed about how to report responsibly. Others spoke more in-depth about a general lack of scientific understanding amongst journalists and the mainstream media particularly when it came to trials, such as in describing participants as 'guinea pigs': 'It was either the BBC or the Guardian that used the word guinea pigs, which obviously is very common. [...] (I)t's not a fair way of describing participants because informed consent is such a massive deal, and we go to such huge lengths to make sure that participants are well informed and understand their rights to withdraw, and all that sort of thing' (Vanderslott, et al. 2021, p. 20). As Dudley et al. (2021) argued, members of the media who focus on science topics should receive specialised training. Some felt that the lack of understanding has contributed to an unrealistic idea of how clinical trials work for the public, which could affect the perception of trial safety. For example, as one participant noted, most people would assume that the vaccine being tested was a live vaccine, and there was nothing to contradict this in the media, corresponding with a sense that the media had an intrinsic lack of scientific understanding: 'the assumption for most people would be that it was the live vaccine' (Patrick-Smith et al. 2024, p. 5).

Participants had a range of views about social media and its role in shaping public perception of the trial. The views fell broadly into two camps: those who thought social media is a vehicle for misinformation, and those who thought it is overall a force for good. One participant felt that social media has had a negative impact on communication about the trial and that there should be no role for it at all. Others commented more on how the information on social media about vaccine trials is untrustworthy, with a participant going as far as to say they did not trust anything that is posted on social media. There was also commentary around how professional some of the misinformation on social media was and how the advent of social media has altered the way misinformation is disseminated. Some had personal experiences of encountering misinformation about the vaccine trial on social media.

One incident that was discussed by multiple participants was the report that the first participant to receive the vaccine had died. This fake news story circulated on social media and was picked up by some more mainstream news outlets before it was shown to be false (*The Guardian* 2020). The story had been about microbiologist Dr Elisa Granato, who woke up on 25 April 2020 to the news that she had died (Image 4.2). Her 'death' had global significance, as she was the first participant in the Oxford-AstraZeneca COVID-19 vaccine trial.

The fake news was widely circulated on social media and was even picked up by some more mainstream news outlets before being shown to be false (*The Guardian* 2020). The viral news across major social media platforms and in the mainstream media fed into concerns that the vaccine was unsafe. Granato had to confirm her 'alive' status on Twitter, however, for many, this rebuttal was even further evidence of a conspiracy that was designed to conceal her death. Such ongoing speculation caused Granato to then release a short video to 'prove' she was still alive, but the authenticity of this was questioned. The Department of Health and Social Care also restated that her death was 'completely untrue' (PA Media 2020).

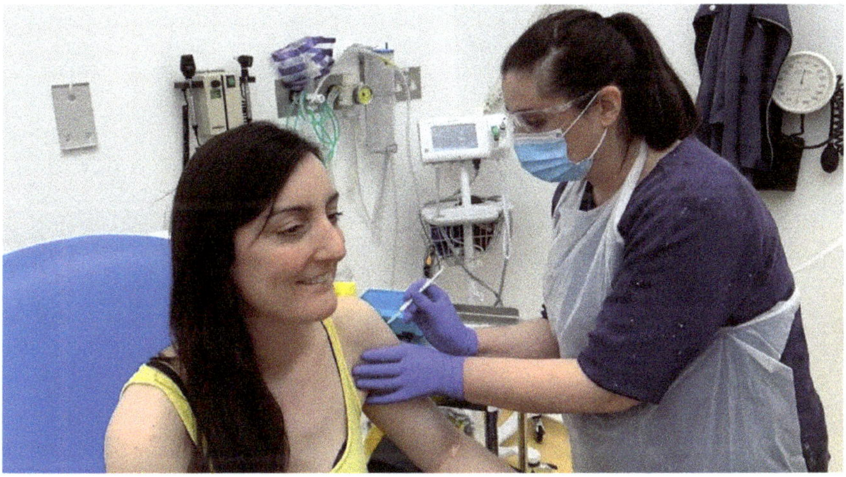

Image 4.2 Elisa Granato, the first participant taking part in the Oxford trial.
Photograph: University of Oxford.

Granato continued to receive messages from those who believed her death was a state-sponsored cover-up months later, adding to the misinformation that undermines confidence in COVID-19 vaccines. Most participants we interviewed who mentioned this story about the first trial participant dying had not believed it at all, although many were concerned about the impact on the trial, with one participant suggesting that it demonstrated the strength of some people's opposition to the vaccine.

Still, social media was felt to be a positive for some participants with the reason that it could be used as a method of educating others about the trial. For instance, a participant spoke of how Twitter had been useful in counteracting fake news and misinformation, having witnessed Twitter users who shared the fake news article being called out by other users: 'I think it's been represented quite well, but I did see one cheeky headline. I think it was The Washington Post the other day who just put a headline out, which is, participant dies in Oxford vaccine trial. And it turns out that

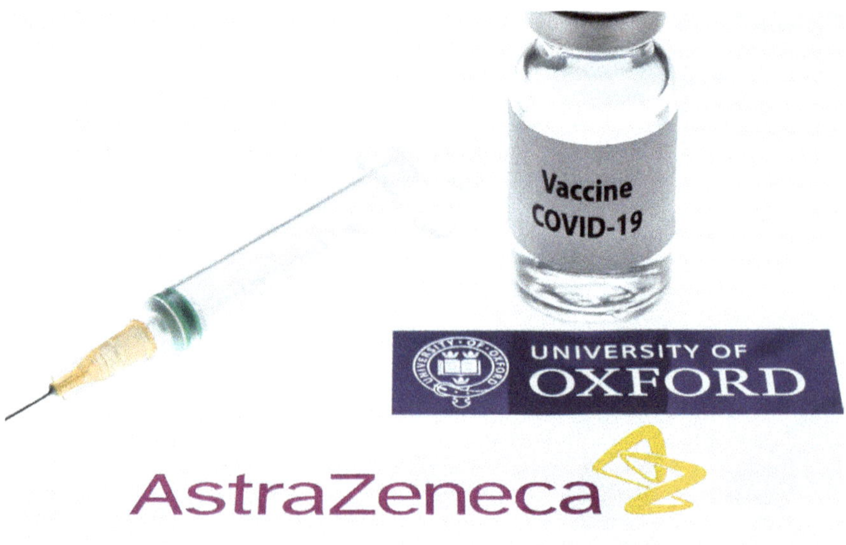

Image 4.3 Oxford-AstraZeneca COVID-19 vaccine.

Photograph: University of Oxford.

he hadn't even had the injection yet or he'd had the placebo or something like that. I think that was represented quite poorly, but I think it was being called out on Twitter for doing that' (Vanderslott et al. 2024, p. 5). Whether social media has the potential to amplify misinformation, therefore, is perhaps dependent on the other users that a person is exposed to, which stands in contrast to the opinion that social media fuels misinformation.

Discussed so far in the chapter have been the roles and responsibilities of the different parties involved in communicating about the Oxford COVID-19 vaccine trial, including the trial participants, trial team, mainstream media, and social media (Image 4.3). Interests and views did not always align between these different parties, and there were some conflicting opinions. Participants were renegotiating their position as being more high profile than usual, and whether that meant they should use this platform or not, which differed depending on the individual. The trial team was viewed as being under a lot of pressure, but participants were generally satisfied with the communication and held a high level of trust in the trial, and especially the principal investigators. In particular, what the media and social media could offer for trial representation was seen in both a positive and negative light.

The final part of this chapter addresses how vaccination is promoted within communities through 'community champions'. This scheme in the United Kingdom utilised volunteers during the COVID-19 pandemic to improve community participation in the vaccination programme – especially amongst groups such as ethnic minorities, who were particularly at risk from COVID-19. This section outlines the background and objectives of the government policy, as well as the challenges and opportunities for community champions.

Community champions

Community volunteers have long been central to health promotion and successful vaccination programmes. This involvement of communities stretches from the participants of vaccine trials to those administering vaccines, although inclusive and wide-ranging community involvement has often been limited to local leaders and elites, such as those with religious authority. Frampton and Shuttleworth (2016) point out that the Global Polio Eradication Initiative, for example, has involved more than 20 million volunteers since it began in 1988, with many working in dangerous conditions. They note how one Somali volunteer, Ali Maow Maalin, was the last person to be infected with naturally occurring smallpox, and after recovering he campaigned for polio eradication (ibid.).

More widely, community engagement has been presented by policymakers, practitioners, and academics as a way to improve access and uptake of health services, including vaccination. Community leaders can be advocates and instrumental in promoting community engagement among ethnic minority groups for vaccination. Health promotion activities have often aimed to also include volunteering programmes that try to work in collaboration with religious and community organisations. These serve as mechanisms to better enable authorities to connect with and tailor support to communities. In particular, earlier research exploring barriers to conducting health research with ethnic minority communities has recommended the deployment of community champions as a solution, as Hood et al. (2015) found in the case of barriers to diabetes research. During the COVID-19 pandemic, a better engagement of at-risk ethnic minority communities was central to the mission of widespread vaccine coverage (Kasstan et al. 2022).

Government policy

A 'Community Champions' scheme was launched by the government in the United Kingdom just prior to the COVID-19 pandemic to develop 'volunteers who, with training and support, help improve the health and wellbeing of their families, communities or workplaces' (gov.uk 2020, p. 1). At the start of 2020, community champions became a focus to aid 'test and trace' policies, with the rationale that such programmes would be useful to address low government trust and provide context-specific solutions to reach vulnerable groups through risk communication and supporting health facilities (ibid.). The Scientific Advisory Group for Emergencies (SAGE) noted that champions needed to be trusted and given autonomy for community participation and to identify activities that meet community needs. Also important was whether there is sincere buy-in from national and local governments, which included proper resourcing to achieve goals. However, it was generally assumed that champions were well equipped to be vaccine promoters and to have the information and expertise needed to answer questions, and not propagate misinformation.

In 2021, the scheme was redirected to support the COVID-19 vaccine roll-out at the community level specifically. The scheme dedicated £23.75 million in funding to 60 councils and voluntary organisations across England, with a focus on 'areas with plans to reach groups such as older people, disabled people, and people from ethnic minority backgrounds' (gov.uk 2021). The focus was on communication and building trust, supporting 'at-risk' groups to share accurate and tailored COVID-19 vaccine advice and health information, as well as tackling misinformation. The overall aim was boosting local vaccination uptake 'and ultimately helping to save lives' via networks of local champions, and by building activities where they already existed (ibid.). Organisations were encouraged to develop their own plans, with activities envisioned as being, for example, 'helplines, school programmes, workplace engagement, phoning those in at risk groups as well as training sessions to help people provide information and advice' (ibid.). The use of phones was suggested for people who might be digitally excluded, to be able also to link them to wider services such as general practitioner (GP) surgeries.

Birmingham was an early example of where support for community champions had been trialled to reach under-served communities across the city (Box 4.5). Birmingham received £440,000 of funding for commissioning helplines and sign language and audio materials for vulnerable groups (e.g. people with learning disabilities, poor literacy, limited digital

Box 4.5 Birmingham community champion case study

'I became a Champion because I'm a childminder. I felt that by being a Champion I could lead by example and ensure that I pass accurate and up-to-date information to other childminders and to the families of the children I care for. I do feel that by following the proper government advice sent through the Community Champion scheme, and with the precautions my work setting put in place, the effect of COVID-19 here has been limited.' (Debbie, aged 52, from Birmingham; gov.uk 2021)

access) to make government guidance more accessible, and to get support for engagement about vaccines through voluntary and community-sector groups (gov.uk 2021). Even though the emphasis in the guidance for the funding had been on using in-person meetings and phones, there was a recognition that virtual communication was needed in a pandemic where social distancing restrictions were in place, and that communities could have a wider reach by utilising social media and online platforms. For example, in some local authorities, community champions shared information from the NHS with local residents via WhatsApp, as well as producing and posting videos of community leaders providing verified information about vaccines via social media (Sussex Health & Care Partnership 2021).

Also, community champions have experienced and confronted the challenges brought on by the pandemic. The COVID-19 pandemic has highlighted both how ethnic minority groups have been disproportionally affected (Mackey et al. 2021) and also the need for community engagement to provide equitable public health information and services (Kadambari and Vanderslott 2021). These community engagement activities and interventions aimed to improve COVID-19 vaccine uptake came against the backdrop of falling vaccination rates more generally (e.g. in 2019 the United Kingdom lost its measles-free status) alongside calls for greater consideration of issues affecting black and minority ethnic groups (e.g. the 'Black Lives Matter' movement). Here also the striking role and influence of media and social media misinformation on vaccine decision making can be seen, especially on black and minority ethnic groups (Zarocostas 2020). However, caution must be exercised in making simplistic assumptions about how misinformation is affecting vaccine uptake negatively in communities, and how a need for well-considered community engagement in a pandemic setting should be addressed.

Hart et al. (2013) specifically consider a community of practice approach for how knowledge is mobilised in partnerships, and how to develop knowledge exchange between diverse actors with differing power hierarchies, such as academics, parents, and practitioners. Understanding how champions view themselves and their positions within wider networks of stakeholders and power differentials is crucial. There are different types of community groups and champions with positions of leadership to take on, creating diversity in what makes a community champion. With colleagues I conducted interviews with community champions to understand the part they play in improving vaccine uptake (Vanderslott et al. 2024). Champions had to consider (1) their target group and the different needs or concerns this entailed (e.g. migrants); (2) the specific vaccine champion role, how they reflect upon that label themselves and how others see them; (3) the importance or impact of champions in their communities, particularly on health inequality (e.g. with wider implications such as routine childhood vaccination); (4) cross-cutting issues, including how ethnic minority classifications are understood, used, and employed through data collection and analysis.

Challenges and opportunities

There were some challenges for community champions that were not well anticipated and complex, requiring more coordination across communities, as well as with health and government organisations. Such issues included how to involve migrants and also people with specific health issues. Many community champions recounted how they worked with migrants, including asylum seekers and refugees as their target group. One champion noted how migrants were worried and fearful about the immigration authorities knowing their whereabouts: '… people living in this way with precarious migration status might not want to interact with the public body due to the hostile environment policies' (ibid. p. 5). The concern was that record keeping and data entry related to a person's vaccine status could make them identifiable by the government, with this information passed onto immigration and border control. Another found that the groups they represent are currently denied many other rights and so have different questions about access to healthcare or might be struggling to access healthcare for vaccines.

A second major issue for champions was the health conditions faced by their target group. One champion worked with people with diabetes, considered as a vulnerable group for COVID-19, as an independent risk factor for severe disease. People of certain ethnicity are more likely to develop type 2 diabetes, which means that they saw lots of people from ethnic minority groups as well.[6] Despite these challenges, considerable weight was placed on the ability of community champions to lead their community on important topics such as vaccination. Reflecting on the vaccine champion role, some of the interviewees did not clearly see the leadership position they held. Champions did not consider themselves to be in positions of leadership but rather of responsibility that had influence, requiring them to act with care (Box 4.6).

A wider challenge was also the difficulty in responding to the needs in communities because of misunderstandings about race and ethnicity, particularly for data and classifications. As one interviewee pointed out, problems arose from broader minority classifications – 'The biggest hurdle was not having accurate ethnicity data' – as well as different local authorities

6 In addition, this champion worked for South Asian Health Foundation, which meant mostly working with minority ethnic groups.

Box 4.6 Quote about community champion leadership

'I don't consider myself to be a leader, as such. I work with local government. I work in the community. And people know me and know me for my sincerity and integrity in what I do. And that I will not actually flout my responsibility. And whatever I say, I won't say it lightly. That's probably the most important thing.' (Vanderslott et al. 2024 p. 5)

and different health boards having different understandings about minority ethnic communities in relation to health and vaccination. The interviewee often found that a comprehensive approach was not taken (Box 4.7).

Despite the challenges, community champions offer opportunities to play an important ongoing vaccination promotion role that could prove especially helpful for future disease outbreaks. This chapter has examined two approaches to fostering public support of vaccination, through communication about vaccines trials, especially by participants, and community champions to promote vaccine rollouts. As demonstrated, determining

Box 4.7 Quote about ethnic minority data and classifications

'There continues to be misunderstandings around race and ethnicity, which, in certain cases, places acronyms on communities, like BAME or BME, which are just not sufficient to respond to the diversity or need within those groups, or very narrow interpretations of legal duties is taken. So, they will just focus on black or South Asian and not on the comprehensive representation of communities and their different health needs. So, there remains a default position to aggregate ethnicities into racial classifications. So, black, white, Asian, other. And we've found them, across the pandemic, just to be utterly useless in terms of identifying individual citizens or community specific needs.' (CC5) roles and responsibilities in such interventions is a crucial activity, and one that is continually evolving. The high expectations placed upon the possibilities of, in particular, online communication and community champions has meant that such activity has been well funded by governments during health crises, such as the COVID-19 pandemic. Indeed, government- and policy-directed initiatives to create communication campaigns, along with ambassadors, role models, and leaders within communities for health objectives, contrasts with the more grassroots activism seen through pro-vaccine activist groups. The trial participants and champions have volunteered their time and efforts to be active online and in their communities, and so specific schemes further facilitate this position. However, to utilise the opportunities presented by champions the sustainability of funding must be guaranteed, which should be available during not only periods of crisis but also in normal times to enable a state of readiness for future pandemics and to address the ongoing health needs of under-served groups in particular.

There are some systemic and deeply rooted challenges in relation to vaccination facing communities that online campaigns, trial participants, and champions cannot be expected to address alone. For example, these included the issue of migrants accessing health services, including vaccination, due to their position and status, the particular health problems that ethnic minorities face, and the availability of relevant race and ethnicity data in order to identify and respond to specific needs. Outside of the COVID-19 pandemic, the potential and limitations of such methods that can encourage or threaten public support deserves the same amount of focus, resourcing, and systemic problem-solving as during a time of crisis.

CHAPTER 5

Conclusion

Vaccination has generally been assumed to be of uncontested public benefit. It has therefore been implemented in health policy through a rational policymaking process, wherein the development, testing, and deployment of vaccines is often undertaken without seriously considering public involvement (addressing potential opposition rather than the potential for public support). Thus, the attention paid to garnering public support for vaccination has been more limited, being characterised by periods of concerted effort, including reactionary responses rather than more dedicated communication and engagement activities. Opposition to vaccination on the other hand has provided the rationale for a focus on how to address the problem of those who are unvaccinated. However, the perceived implication has been that there is no need to turn to those who vaccinate and display active support, or investigate how to best foster and encourage this demographic.

This book has concentrated on the interplay between civil society advocacy and public stakeholders, with activities such as activism, petitions, and trials within the contentious realm of vaccination across different times and places. Such a variation in examples suggests that support for vaccines is a fragile and ongoing effort. It is an effort that relies on trust and confidence in governments and public policy, universities and pharmaceutical companies, scientists, regulators, health institutions, and healthcare workers, as well as positive representations on social and mainstream media. Public agreement with institutions and actors related to areas of the personal sphere such as healthcare and parenting is far from unanimous. Suspicion and mistrust are increasing towards experts and large multinational companies, particularly 'big pharma', philanthropic organisations, as well as international health institutions like the World Health Organization (WHO). Indeed, there are also credible or legitimate reasons for lack of trust in different historical and geographic contexts.

To shed light on how vaccination is supported in society, I have explored case studies of various vaccination campaigns, showing the role of advocacy and activism in bringing health issues to the attention of the public, media, and policymakers. These cases have explored how support for vaccine-preventable diseases (meningitis, measles and pertussis, typhoid fever, COVID-19) and the influence of vaccine policies and public attitudes, are deeply rooted and profoundly felt for a medical intervention that has had widespread social implications. By focusing on a pro-vaccine perspective, I have situated such views and actions within a dynamic landscape that also includes those who oppose vaccines, and public policies that range from mildly encouraging to coercively mandating vaccination. While pro-vaccine stories may not receive as much coverage as their counterparts, the narratives and associated activist campaigns have gained some prominence, and my aim has been to balance the discussion by analysing these activities. This book therefore reveals the diverse forms that pro-vaccine views and behaviours can take, and pro-vaccine involvement in vaccine development, trials, and policies to encourage or compel vaccination against vaccine-preventable diseases, including the impact of political economy, philanthropy, and the media in particular. Such a focus challenges the prevailing notion of growing opposition and scepticism among vaccinating populations, further amplified by an anti-vaccine minority. The depiction of a polarised, camp-based, oppositional arena is more nuanced and complex in reality. In fact, pro-vaccine support is much more active and varied than might be assumed and in comparison to what is viewed to be a forceful and effective anti-vaccine lobby.

In providing a better understanding of pro-vaccine actors and activities I have aimed to reveal how and why support happens, how it can be sustained, and what can be done to foster support and address its waning or absence. This support for vaccination is multifaceted and contains contradictions as well as the need to balance competing priorities. It is highly dependent on context, varies across countries, time, and particular diseases or vaccines, and depends on the individual actors and groups involved. Sustaining vaccine support is also done against the backdrop of both outbreaks and ongoing public and community engagement. Further, I have suggested potential new avenues to foster vaccine support online, through trial participants on social and mainstream media, as well as through community champions taking a continued role.

It is clear that the scientific and public health success of vaccine development alone is not sufficient. While vaccines must be produced safely at scale, with efficient rollout – a population ready and willing to be vaccinated is a core requirement too – and remains an ongoing question of relationship-building and trust between many different stakeholders. Support for vaccination will continue to be intertwined with geopolitical and socio-economic factors – such factors significantly influence which populations, both within and across national borders, benefit the most from vaccines. Disparities are present nationally, in health outcomes as well as in vaccine uptake; and internationally, where for example during the COVID-19 pandemic, those who secured the best supply deals with pharmaceutical companies fared better in their access. However, vaccine nationalism and staggering vaccine inequity worldwide, whilst improving on some fronts, still remain persistent issues for improved vaccine uptake and thus global health generally. In conjunction, for comprehensive vaccine protection worldwide to be achieved, better arrangements are also needed to ensure sufficient public acceptance and uptake in the face of inevitable future pandemics: drawing on public support of vaccination should be a important piece of this puzzle.

Bibliography

Abeysinghe, Sudeepa. 2015. 'Vaccine Narratives and Public Health: Investigating Criticisms of H1N1 Pandemic Vaccination'. *PLoS Currents*. Feb 25; 7: <https://doi:10.1371/currents.outbreaks.17b6007099e92486483872ff39ede178>.

Aggett, Siân. 2018. 'Turning the Gaze: Challenges of Involving Biomedical Researchers in Community Engagement with Research in Patan, Nepal'. *Critical Public Health* 28 (3): 306–17. <https://doi.org/10.1080/09581596.2018.1443203>.

Almond, Jeffrey, Jörg Hacker, Colin Harwood, Mariagrazia Pizza, Rino Rappuoli, Eliora Z. Ron, Philippe Sansonetti, Samantha Vanderslott, and Lothar H. Wieler. 2020. 'Development of Vaccines at the Time of COVID-19'. *MicroLife* 1 (1). <https://doi.org/10.1093/femsml/uqaa003>.

Al-Shehri, Sulieman N., and Sulaiman A. Al-Shammari. 1991. 'Immunization Coverage Survey in Eight Regions of Saudi Arabia'. *Annals of Tropical Paediatrics* 11 (2): 181–7. <https://doi.org/10.1080/02724936.1991.11747499>.

American Academy of Pediatrics. 2011. 'Meningococcal Conjugate Vaccines Policy Update: Booster Dose Recommendations'. *Pediatrics* 128 (6): 1212–9. <https://doi.org/ 10.1542/peds.2011-2380>.

Ames, Heather M. R., Claire Glenton, and Simon Lewin. 2017. 'Parents' and Informal Caregivers' Views and Experiences of Communication about Routine Childhood Vaccination: A Synthesis of Qualitative Evidence'. *The Cochrane Database of Systematic Reviews* 2 (2): 1–121. <https://doi.org/10.1002/14651858.CD011787.PUB2>.

Amodio, Emanuele, Francesco Vitale, Livia Cimino, Alessandra Casuccio, and Fabio Tramuto. 2020. 'Outbreak of Novel Coronavirus (SARS-CoV-2): First Evidences from International Scientific Literature and Pending Questions'. *Healthcare* 8 (1): 51. <https://doi.org/10.3390/healthcare8010051>.

Anderson, Edward, and Christophe Jaffrelot. 2018. 'Hindu Nationalism and the 'Saffronisation of the Public Sphere': An Interview with Christophe Jaffrelot'. *Contemporary South Asia* 26 (4): 468–82. <https://doi.org/10.1080/09584935.2018.1545009>.

Andrews, Sophie M., and Andrew J. Pollard. 2014. 'A Vaccine against Serogroup B *Neisseria Meningitidis*: Dealing with Uncertainty'. *The Lancet Infectious Diseases* 14 (5): 426–34. <https://doi.org/10.1016/S1473-3099(13)70341-4>.

Anheier, Helmut K. 2013. *Civil Society: Measurement, Evaluation, Policy*. London: Routledge.

Armstrong, Gregory L., Laura A. Conn, and Robert W. Pinner. 1999. 'Trends in Infectious Disease Mortality in the United States during the 20th Century'. *JAMA* 281 (1): 61–6. <https://doi.org/10.1001/JAMA.281.1.61>.

Attwell, Katie, and David T. Smith. 2017. 'Parenting as Politics: Social Identity Theory and Vaccine Hesitant Communities'. *International Journal of Health Governance* 22 (3): 183–98. <https://doi.org/10.1108/IJHG-03-2017-0008>.

Attwell, Katie, Adam Hannah, and Julie Leask. 2022. 'COVID-19: Talk of 'Vaccine Hesitancy' Lets Governments Off the Hook'. *Nature* 602 (7898): 574–7. <https://doi.org/10.1038/d41586-022-00495-8>.

Baker, Jeffrey P., and Samuel L. Katz. 2004. 'Childhood Vaccine Development: An Overview'. *Pediatric Research* 55 (2): 347–56. <https://doi.org/10.1203/01.pdr.0000106317.36875.6a>.

Barber, Sarah. 2016. 'Meningitis B Vaccination'. House of Commons Library. <https://commonslibrary.parliament.uk/research-briefings/cbp-7569/>.

Bateman-House, Alison. 2009. 'Men of peace and the search for the perfect pesticide: Conscientious objectors, the Rockefeller Foundation, and typhus control research'. *Public Health Reports* 124(4), pp.594–602. <https://doi.org/10.1177/003335490912400418>.

Baylac-Paouly, Baptiste. 2019. 'Vaccine Development as a "Doable Problem": The Case of the Meningococcal A Vaccines 1962–1969'. *Studies in History and Philosophy of Science Part C: Studies in History and Philosophy of Biological and Biomedical Sciences* 74 (April): 7–14. <https://doi.org/10.1016/J.SHPSC.2019.01.001>.

BBC News. 1990. 'Typhoid Women Were Kept in Asylum.' <http://news.bbc.co.uk/2/hi/uk_news/7528045.stm>.

BBC News. 2013a. 'Meningitis Trust and Meningitis UK to Merge.' <https://www.bbc.co.uk/news/uk-england-gloucestershire-21798630>.

BBC News. 2013b. 'Swansea Measles Epidemic Officially Over.' <https://www.bbc.com/news/uk-wales-23168519>.

BBC News. 2018. 'Council Backs Move to Stop Anti-abortion "Harassment" – BBC News'. <https://www.bbc.co.uk/news/uk-england-manchester-42804751>.

Beard, Frank H., Julie Leask, and Peter B. McIntyre. 2017. 'No Jab, No Pay and Vaccine Refusal in Australia: The Jury Is Out.' *The Medical Journal of Australia* 206 (9): 381–83. <https://doi.org/10.5694/mja16.00944>.

Bedford, Helen, Katie Attwell, Margie Danchin, Helen Marshall, Paul Corben, and Julie Leask. 2018. 'Vaccine Hesitancy, Refusal and Access Barriers: The Need for Clarity in Terminology'. *Vaccine* 36 (44): 6556–58. <https://doi.org/10.1016/J.VACCINE.2017.08.004>.

Bednarczyk, Robert. A. 2015. 'Human papillomavirus vaccine and sexual activity: How do we best address parent and physician concerns?'. *JAMA Intern Med* 175 (4): 624–625. <https://doi.org/10.1001/jamainternmed.2014.7894>.

Beebee, Helen. 2018. 'I – The Presidential Address Philosophical Scepticism and the Aims of Philosophy'. *Proceedings of the Aristotelian Society* 118 (1): 1–24. <https://doi.org/10.1093/ARISOC/AOX017>.

Benford, Robert D. 1993. '"You Could Be the Hundredth Monkey": Collective Action Frames and Vocabularies of Motive within the Nuclear Disarmament Movement'. *Sociological Quarterly* 34 (2): 195–216. <https://doi.org/10.1111/j.1533-8525.1993.tb00387.x>.

Bennett, Joan W., and King Thom Chung. 2001. 'Alexander Fleming and the Discovery of Penicillin'. *Advances in Applied Microbiology* 49 (January): 163–84. <https://doi.org/10.1016/S0065-2164(01)49013-7>.

Betsch, Cornelia, Philipp Schmid, Dorothee Heinemeier, Lars Korn, Cindy Holtmann, and Robert Böhm. 2018. 'Beyond Confidence: Development of a Measure Assessing the 5C Psychological Antecedents of Vaccination'. *PLoS ONE* 13 (12). <https://doi.org/10.1371/JOURNAL.PONE.0208601>.

Bhattacharya, Sanjoy, and Carlos Eduardo D'Avila Pereira Campani. 2020. 'Re-assessing the Foundations: Worldwide Smallpox Eradication, 1957–67'. *Medical History* 64 (1): 71–93. <https://doi.org/10.1017/MDH.2019.77>.

Bloom, David E., Daniel Cadarette, Maddalena Ferranna, Randall N. Hyer, and Daniel L. Tortorice. 2021. 'How New Models of Vaccine Development for COVID-19 Have Helped Address an Epic Public Health Crisis'. *Health Affairs* 40 (3): 410–18. <https://doi.org/10.1377/hlthaff.2020.02012>.

Bloor, David. 1991. *Knowledge and Social Imagery*. Chicago: University of Chicago Press.

Blume, Stuart. 2006. 'Anti-vaccination Movements and Their Interpretations.' *Social Science & Medicine* 62 (3): 628–42. <https://doi.org/10.1016/j.socscimed.2005.06.020>.

Blume, Stuart, Christine Holmberg, and Paul R. Greenough. 2017. *The Politics of Vaccination: A Global History*. Manchester University Press: Manchester.

Blume, Stuart. 2017. *Immunization: How Vaccines Became Controversial*. London: Reaktion Books.

Bramwell, Neil. 2014. 'Not Qualified to Speak Out?' *Medical Observer*. <https://www.medicalobserver.com.au/professional-news/not-qualified-to-speak-out>.

Brehony, Carina, Dorothea M. Hill, Jay, Lucidarme, Ray Borrow, and Martin. C. Maiden. 2015. 'Meningococcal Vaccine Antigen Diversity in Global Databases'. *Eurosurveillance* 20 (49): 1–9. <https://doi.org/10.2807/1560-7917.ES.2015.20.49.30084>.

Brown, Phil, and Stephen Zavestoski. 2004. 'Social Movements in Health: An Introduction.' *Sociology of Health and Illness* 26 (6): 679–94. <https://doi.org/10.1111/j.0141-9889.2004.00413.x>.

Brown, Phil, Stephen Zavestoski, Sabrina McCormick, Brian Mayer, Rachel Morello-Frosch, and Rebecca Gasior Altman. 2004. 'Embodied Health Movements: New Approaches to Social Movements in Health.' *Sociology of Health and Illness* 26 (1): 50–80. <https://doi.org/10.1111/j.1467-9566.2004.00378.x>.

Browne, Matthew. 2018. 'Epistemic Divides and Ontological Confusions: The Psychology of Vaccine Scepticism'. *Human Vaccines & Immunotherapeutics* 14 (10): 2540–42. <https://doi.org/10.1080/21645515.2018.1480244>.

Browne, Sarah, Tarweh Carter, Risa Eckes, Greg Grandits, Melvin Johnson, Irene Moore, and Laura McNay. 2018. 'A Review of Strategies Used to Retain Participants in Clinical Research during an Infectious Disease Outbreak: The PREVAIL I Ebola Vaccine Trial Experience'. *Contemporary Clinical Trials Communications* 11 (September): 50–54. <https://doi.org/10.1016/J.CONCTC.2018.06.004>.

Brunson, Emily K., and Elisa J. Sobo. 2017. 'Framing Childhood Vaccination in the United States: Getting Past Polarization in the Public Discourse'. *Human Organization* 76 (1): 38–47. <https://doi.org/10.17730/0018-7259.76.1.38>.

Buchanan, Mark. 2020. 'Managing the Infodemic'. *Nature Physics* 16: 894. <https://doi.org/10.1038/s41567-020-01039-5>.

Bufacchi, Vittorio. 2022. 'Mandatory Vaccination Not the Same as Compulsory.' *Irish Times*. <https://www.irishtimes.com/opinion/mandatory-vaccination-not-the-same-as-compulsory-1.4774909>.

Burgess, Rochelle Ann, Richard H. Osborne, Kenneth A. Yongabi, Trisha Greenhalgh, Deepti Gurdasani, Gagandeep Kang, Adegoke G. Falade, Rochelle Ann Burgess, Richard H Osborne, Kenneth A Yongabi, Trisha Greenhalgh, Deepti Gurdasani, Gagandeep Kang, Adegoke G Falade, Anna Odone, Reinhard Busse, Jose M Martin-Moreno, Stephen Reicher, Martin McKee. 2021. 'The COVID-19 Vaccines Rush: Participatory Community Engagement Matters More than Ever.' *Lancet* 397 (10268): 8–10. <https://doi.org/10.1016/S0140-6736(20)32642-8>.

Burki, Talha. 2020. 'The Online Anti-vaccine Movement in the Age of COVID-19.' *Lancet Digital Health* 2 (10): e504–5. <https://doi.org/10.1016/S2589-7500(20)30227-2>.

Busby, Colin, Aaron Jacobs, and Ramya Muthukumaran. 2017. 'In Need of a Booster: How to Improve Childhood Vaccination Coverage in Canada (Besoin D'Un Rappel? Comment Améliorer La Couverture Vaccinale Des

Enfants AU Canada)'. *SSRN Electronic Journal*, April. <https://doi.org/10.2139/SSRN.2962393>.

Butt, Muhammad Hammad, Aqsa Saleem, Syed Owais Javed, Irfan Ullah, Mujeeb Ur Rehman, Nayyer Islam, Muhammad Azam Tahir, Tangina Malik, Sara Hafeez, and Shahzadi Misbah. 2022. 'Rising XDR-Typhoid Fever Cases in Pakistan: Are We Heading Back to the Pre-antibiotic Era?' *Frontiers in Public Health* 9 (January): 2049. <https://doi.org/10.3389/fpubh.2021.794868>.

Calina, Daniela, Thomas Hartung, Anca Oana Docea, Demetrios A. Spandidos, Alex M. Egorov, Michael I. Shtilman, Felix Carvalho, and Aristidis Tsatsakis. 2020. 'COVID-19 Vaccines: Ethical Framework Concerning Human Challenge Studies'. *DARU, Journal of Pharmaceutical Sciences* 28 (2): 807–12. <https://doi.org/10.1007/s40199-020-00371-8>.

Callis, Amy, Victoria M. Carter, Aparna Ramakrishnan, Alison P. Albert, Lansana Conteh, Alhaji Amadu Barrie, Lucian Fahnbulleh, Amy Callis, Victoria M Carter, Aparna Ramakrishnan, Alison P Albert, Lansana Conteh, Alhaji Amadu Barrie, Lucian Fahnbulleh, Mark M Koroma, Samuel Saidu, Otis Williams, and Mohamed Samai. 2018. 'Lessons Learned in Clinical Trial Communication During an Ebola Outbreak: The Implementation of STRIVE'. *Journal of Infectious Diseases* 217 (suppl. 1): S40–47. <https://doi.org/10.1093/INFDIS/JIX558>.

Carey, Megan E., Zoey I. Diaz, Martin Broadstock, Roderick Bailey, Adwoa D. Bentsi-Enchill, and Heidi J Larson. 2019. 'Toward Control? The Prospects and Challenges of Typhoid Conjugate Vaccine Introduction.' *Clinical Infectious Diseases* 69 (suppl. 5): S408–11. <https://doi.org/10.1093/cid/ciz483>.

CDC. n.d. 'Immunization Basics'. Accessed February 27, 2024. <https://www.cdc.gov/vaccines/vac-gen/imz-basics.htm#>.

Change.org. n.d. 'Eliminate the "Personal Belief" Vaccine Exemption That's Putting Sick California Kids at Risk'. Accessed 27 May 2018. <https://www.change.org/p/california-governor-eliminate-the-personal-belief-vaccine-exemption-that-s-putting-sick-california-kids-at-risk>.

Christensen, Hannah, Caroline L. Trotter, Matthew Hickman, and W. John Edmunds. 2014. 'Re-evaluating Cost Effectiveness of Universal Meningitis Vaccination (Bexsero) in England: Modelling Study'. *BMJ* 349 (October). <https://doi.org/10.1136/BMJ.G5725>.

CIDRAP and the Wellcome Trust. 2015. 'Recommendations for Accelerating the Development of Ebola Vaccines'. <http://www.cidrap.umn.edu/recommendations-accelerating-development-ebola-vaccines-0>.

Clark, Ann. 2004. 'Compliance with Infant Smallpox Vaccination Legislation in Nineteenth-Century Rural England: Hollingbourne, 1876–88'. *Social History of Medicine* 17 (2): 175–98. <https://doi.org/10.1093/SHM/17.2.175>.

Cohen, Jon. 2016. 'The Truest Test'. *Science* 352 (6288): 882–5. <https://www.science.org/doi/10.1126/science.352.6288.882>.

Comfort, Nathaniel. 2009. 'The Prisoner as Model Organism: Malaria Research at Stateville Penitentiary'. *Studies in History and Philosophy of Biological and Biomedical Sciences* 40 (3): 190. <https://doi.org/10.1016/J.shpsc.2009.06.007>.

Conis, Elena. 2015. *Vaccine Nation : America's Changing Relationship with Immunization*. 1st ed. Chicago: University of Chicago Press.

Cookson, Clive. 2020. 'Sarah Gilbert, the Researcher Leading the Race to a Covid-19 Vaccine'. *Financial Times*. <https://www.ft.com/content/d2ae1fff-9747-41a3-b347-861ac1a70709>.

COVID-19 Oxford Vaccine Trial. n.d. 'Participate Birmingham'. Accessed 19 March 2021. <https://covid19vaccinetrial.co.uk/participate-birmingham>.

Cyranoski, David. 2019. 'The CRISPR-Baby Scandal: What's Next for Human Gene-Editing'. *Nature* 566 (7745): 440–2. <https://doi.org/10.1038/D41586-019-00673-1>.

Darton, Thomas C., Christoph J. Blohmke, Vasee S. Moorthy, Daniel M. Altmann, Frederick G. Hayden, Elizabeth A. Clutterbuck, Myron M. Levine, Adrian V.S. Hill, and Andrew J. Pollard. 2015. 'Design, Recruitment, and Microbiological Considerations in Human Challenge Studies'. *Lancet. Infectious Diseases* 15 (7): 840–51. <https://doi.org/10.1016/S1473-3099(15)00068-7>.

Deer, Brian. 2011. 'How the Case against the MMR Vaccine Was Fixed'. *BMJ* 342 (7788): 77–82. <https://doi.org/10.1136/BMJ.C5347>.

Department of Health and Social Care Media Centre. 2016. 'Jane Ellison, Public Health Minister, Announces New Public Awareness Campaign for Meningitis, Sepsis and Septicaemia'. DH Media Centre. <https://healthmedia.blog.gov.uk/2016/04/26/jane-ellison-public-health-minister-announces-new-public-awareness-campaign-for-meningitis-sepsis-and-septicaemia/>.

Detoc, Maelle, Amandine Gagneux-Brunon, Frédéric Lucht, and Elisabeth Botelho-Nevers. 2017. 'Barriers and Motivations to Volunteers' Participation in Preventive Vaccine Trials: A Systematic Review'. *Expert Review of Vaccines* 16 (5): 467–77. <https://doi.org/10.1080/14760584.2017.1297706>.

Detoc, Maelle, Odile Launay, Christian Dualé, Catherine Mutter, Jean-Charles Le Huec, Nezha Lenzi, Frédéric Lucht, Amandine Gagneux-Brunon, and Elisabeth Botelho-Nevers. 2019. 'Barriers and Motivations for Participation in Preventive Vaccine Clinical Trials: Experience of 5 Clinical Research Sites'. *Vaccine* 37 (44): 6633–9. <https://doi.org/10.1016/J.VACCINE.2019.09.048>.

Dhalla, Shayesta, and Gary Poole. 2011. 'Motivators of Enrolment in HIV Vaccine Trials: A Review of HIV Vaccine Preparedness Studies'. *AIDS Care* 23 (11): 1430–47. <https://doi.org/10.1080/09540121.2011.555750>.

DiResta, Renee. 2017. 'This Dramatic Graph Shows How the Pro-vaccine Movement Can Win'. *Slate*, April. <http://www.slate.com/articles/health_and_science/medical_examiner/2017/04/this_dramatic_graph_shows_how_the_pro_vaccine_movement_can_win.html>.

Dixon, Justin, and Michèle Tameris. 2018. 'Clean Blood, Religion, and Moral Triage in Tuberculosis Vaccine Trials'. *Medical Anthropology: Cross Cultural Studies in Health and Illness* 37 (8): 708–21. <https://doi.org/10.1080/01459740.2018.1463528>.

Doshi, Sucheta, Nino Khetsuriani, Khatuna Zakhashvili, Levan Baidoshvili, Paata Imnadze, and Amra Uzicanin. 2009. 'Ongoing Measles and Rubella Transmission in Georgia, 2004–05: Implications for the National and Regional Elimination Efforts'. *International Journal of Epidemiology* 38 (1): 182–91. <https://doi.org/10.1093/IJE/DYN261>.

Dubé, Eve, Dominique Gagnon, Noni E. MacDonald, the SAGE Working Group on Vaccine Hesitancy 2015. 'Strategies Intended to Address Vaccine Hesitancy: Review of Published Reviews'. *Vaccine* 33 (34): 4191–203. <https://doi.org/10.1016/J.VACCINE.2015.04.041>.

Dubé, Eve, Caroline Laberge, Maryse Guay, Paul Bramadat, Réal Roy, and Julie Bettinger. 2013. 'Vaccine Hesitancy: An Overview'. *Human Vaccines & Immunotherapeutics* 9 (8): 1763–73. <https://doi.org/10.4161/HV.24657>.

Dubé, Ève, Jeremy K. Ward, Pierre Verger, and Noni E. Macdonald. 2021. 'Vaccine Hesitancy, Acceptance, and Anti-vaccination: Trends and Future Prospects for Public Health'. *Annual Review of Public Health* 42 (April): 175–91. <https://doi.org/10.1146/ANNUREV-PUBLHEALTH-090419-102240>.

Dudley, Matthew Z., Roger Bernier, Janesse Brewer, and Daniel A. Salmon. 2021. 'Walking the Tightrope: Reevaluating Science Communication in the Era of COVID-19 Vaccines'. *Vaccine* 39 (39): 5453–5. <https://doi.org/10.1016/J.vaccine.2021.08.037>.

Dunlop, Rachael. 2013a. 'A View on Vaccination Myths'. *Conversation*. <https://theconversation.com/a-view-on-vaccination-myths-14699>.

Dunlop, Rachael. 2013b. 'Anti-vaccination Activists Should Not Be Given a Say in the Media'. *Guardian*. <https://www.theguardian.com/commentisfree/2013/oct/16/anti-vaccination-activists-should-not-be-given-a-say-in-the-media>.

Durbach, Nadja. 2004. *Bodily Matters: The Anti-vaccination Movement in England, 1853–1907*. 1–276. Durham NC/London:Duke University Press.

Dutta, Tapati, Jon Agley, Beth E. Meyerson, Priscilla A. Barnes, Catherine Sherwood-Laughlin, and Jill Nicholson-Crotty. 2021. 'Perceived Enablers and Barriers of Community Engagement for Vaccination in India: Using Socioecological Analysis'. *PLOS ONE* 16 (6): e0253318. <https://doi.org/10.1371/JOURNAL.PONE.0253318>.

Ellenberg, Susan S. 2020. 'Clinical Trials in the Time of a Pandemic'. *Clinical Trials* 17 (5): 467–71. <https://doi.org/10.1177/1740774520939871>.

Ellerton, Peter. 2014. 'The Problem of False Balance When Reporting on Science'. *Conversation.* <https://theconversation.com/the-problem-of-false-balance-when-reporting-on-science-29077>.

Elliott, Carl, and Roberto Abadie. 2009. 'Exploiting a Research Underclass in Phase 1 Clinical Trials'. *The New England Journal of Medicine* 358 (22): 2316–17. <https://doi.org/10.1056/NEJMP0801872>.

Epps, Heather L. Van. 2006. 'René Dubos: Unearthing Antibiotics'. *Journal of Experimental Medicine* 203 (2): 259. <https://doi.org/10.1084/JEM.2032FTA>.

Esveld, Marja. 2002. 'Dutch Initiate Major Vaccination Campaign against Meningitis C'. *Eurosurveillance* 6 (18): 1–2128. <https://doi.org/10.2807/ESW.06.18.02128-EN>.

Eyal, Nir, Marc Lipsitch, and Peter G. Smith. 2020. 'Human Challenge Studies to Accelerate Coronavirus Vaccine Licensure'. *Journal of Infectious Diseases* 221 (11): 1752. <https://doi.org/10.1093/INFDIS/JIAA152>.

Faasse, Kate, Casey J. Chatman, and Leslie R. Martin. 2016. 'A Comparison of Language Use in Pro- and Anti-vaccination Comments in Response to a High Profile Facebook Post'. *Vaccine* 34 (47): 5808–14. <https://doi.org/10.1016/J.VACCINE.2016.09.029>.

Favin, Michael, Robert Steinglass, Rebecca Fields, Kaushik Banerjee, and Monika Sawhney. 2012. 'Why Children Are Not Vaccinated: A Review of the Grey Literature'. *International Health* 4 (4): 229–38. <https://doi.org/10.1016/J.INHE.2012.07.004>.

Figueiredo, Alex de, Rachel. L. Eagan, Greet Hendrickx, Emilie Karafillakis, Pierre Van Damme, and Heidi J. Larson. 2022. State of Vaccine Confidence in the European Union 2022. Luxembourg: Publications Office of the European Union. 31–2. <https:// doi.org/ 10.2875/ 188 426>.

Finn, Patrick, Anne K. Bothe, and Robin E. Bramlett. 2005. 'Science and Pseudoscience in Communication Disorders'. *American Journal of Speech-Language Pathology* 14 (3): 172–86. <https://doi.org/10.1044/1058-0360(2005/018)>.

Finnegan, Gary, Daphne Holt, Peter M. English, Steffen Glismann, Angus Thomson, David M. Salisbury, Hugues Bogaerts, and Paolo Bonanni. 2018. 'Lessons from an Online Vaccine Communication Project'. *Vaccine* 36 (44): 6509–11. <https://doi.org/10.1016/J.vaccine.2018.05.007>.

Fisher, Jill A. 2020. *Adverse Events: Race, Inequality, and the Testing of New Pharmaceuticals*. New York: New York University Press.

Fitzpatrick, Michael. 2008. 'Medicine and the Media: From Hero to Zero'. *BMJ* 336 (7642): 479. <https://doi.org/10.1136/BMJ.39492.664225.0F>.

Folegatti, Pedro M., Katie J. Ewer, Parvinder K. Aley, Brian Angus, Stephan Becker, Sandra Belij-Rammerstorfer, Duncan Bellamy, et al. 2020. 'Safety and Immunogenicity of the ChAdOx1 NCoV-19 Vaccine against SARS-CoV-2: A Preliminary Report of a Phase 1/2, Single-Blind, Randomised Controlled Trial'. *Lancet* 396 (10249): 467–78. <https://doi.org/10.1016/S0140-6736(20)31604-4>.

Fonseca, Elize M. da, Holly Jarman, Elizabeth J. King, and Scott L. Greer. 2022. 'Perspectives in the study of the political economy of COVID–19 vaccine regulation.' *Regulation & Governance* 16, no. 4: 1283–1289. <https://doi.org/10.1111/rego.12413>.

Fragkaki, Iro, Dominique F. Maciejewski, Esther L. Weijman, Jonas Feltes, and Maaike Cima. 2021. 'Human Responses to Covid-19: The Role of Optimism Bias, Perceived Severity, and Anxiety'. *Personality and Individual Differences* 176 (July): 110781. <https://doi.org/10.1016/J.PAID.2021.110781>.

Frampton, Sally, and Sally Shuttleworth. 2016. 'Medical Research: Citizen Medicine'. *Nature* 534 (7607): 324–324. <https://doi.org/10.1038/534324a>.

Freedman, David O., Abinash Virk, and Elaine C. Jong. 2008. 'Immunization of Healthy Adults'. *Travel Medicine: Second Edition*, June, 85–120. <https://doi.org/10.1016/B978-0-323-03453-1.10010-0>.

Garrett, Denise O., Ashley T. Longley, Kristen Aiemjoy, Mohammad T. Yousafzai, Caitlin Hemlock, Alexander T. Yu, Krista Vaidya, et al. 2022. 'Incidence of Typhoid and Paratyphoid Fever in Bangladesh, Nepal, and Pakistan: Results of the Surveillance for Enteric Fever in Asia Project'. *Lancet Global Health* 10 (7): e978–88. <https://doi.org/10.1016/S2214-109X(22)00119-X>.

Geest, Sjaak van der, and Susan Reynolds Whyte. 1989. 'The Charm of Medicines: Metaphors and Metonyms'. *Medical Anthropology Quarterly* 3 (4): 345–67. <https://doi.org/10.1525/maq.1989.3.4.02a00030>.

Gilbert, Sarah, Catherine Green, and Deborah Crewe. 2021. *Vaxxers: The Inside Story of the Oxford AstraZeneca Vaccine and the Race against the Virus*. London: Hodder & Stoughton.

Girard, Marc P., Marie Pierre Preziosi, Maria Teresa Aguado, and Marie Paule Kieny. 2006. 'A Review of Vaccine Research and Development: Meningococcal Disease'. *Vaccine* 24 (22): 4692–700. <https://doi.org/10.1016/J.VACCINE.2006.03.034>.

Giubilini, Alberto. 2019. 'Vaccination Policies and the Principle of Least Restrictive Alternative: An Intervention Ladder'. *Ethics of Vaccination*, 59–93. Basingstoke: Springer Nature <https://doi.org/10.1007/978-3-030-02068-2_3>.

Giubilini, Alberto, and Julian Savulescu. 2019. 'Demandingness and Public Health Ethics'. *Moral Philosophy and Politics* 6 (1): 65–87. <https://doi.org/10.1044/1058-0360(2005/018)>.

Godlee, Fiona, Jane Smith, and Harvey Marcovitch. 2011. 'Wakefield's Article Linking MMR Vaccine and Autism Was Fraudulent'. *BMJ* 342 (7788): 64–6. <https://doi.org/10.1136/bmj.C7452>.

Goodwin, Jeff, James M. Jasper, Myra Marx Ferree, Richard Flacks, Marshall Ganz, Jeff Goodwin, Deborah B. Gould, Jeff Goodwin and James M. Jasper (Editors). 2003. *Rethinking Social Movements : Structure, Meaning, and Emotion.* Maryland: Rowman & Littlefield Publishers.

gov.uk. 2015. 'Meningococcal B: Vaccine Information for Healthcare Professionals'. 3 July. <https://webarchive.nationalarchives.gov.uk/ukgwa/20150711130355/https://www.gov.uk/government/publications/meningococcal-b-vaccine-information-for-healthcare-professionals>.

gov.uk. 2020. 'Role of Community Champions Networks to Increase Engagement in Context of COVID-19: Evidence and Best Practice, 22 October 2020'. 6 November. <https://www.gov.uk/government/publications/role-of-commun ity-champions-networks-to-increase-engagement-in-context-of-covid-19-evidence-and-best-practice-22-october-2020>.

gov.uk. 2021. 'Community Champions to Give COVID-19 Vaccine Advice and Boost Take up – gov.uk'. 25 January. <https://www.gov.uk/government/news/community-champions-to-give-covid-19-vaccine-advice-and-boost-take-up>.

gov.uk. 2022. 'UK Measles and Rubella Elimination Indicators and Status'. 23 November. <https://www.gov.uk/government/publications/measles-and-rubella-elimination-uk/uk-measles-and-rubella-elimination#:~:text=The%20WHO%20confirmed%20that%20the,established%20transmission%20of%20measles%20virus>.

Gradmann, Christoph. 2010. 'Robert Koch and the Invention of the Carrier State: Tropical Medicine, Veterinary Infections and Epidemiology around 1900'. *Studies in History and Philosophy of Biological and Biomedical Sciences* 41 (3): 232–40. <https://doi.org/10.1016/J.SHPSC.2010.04.012>.

Gradmann, Christoph, Mark Harrison, and Anne Rasmussen. 2019. 'Typhoid and the Military in the Early 20th Century'. *Clinical Infectious Diseases* 69 (5): S385–87. <https://doi.org/10.1093/cid/ciz672>.

Grandahl, Maria, Marie Oscarsson, Christina Stenhammar, Tryggve Nevéus, Ragnar Westerling, and Tanja Tydén. 2014. 'Not the Right Time: Why Parents Refuse to Let Their Daughters Have the Human Papillomavirus Vaccination'. *Acta Paediatrica* 103 (4): 436–41. <https://doi.org/10.1111/APA.12545>.

Grant, Lenny, Bernice L. Hausman, Margaret Cashion, Nicholas Lucchesi, Kelsey Patel, and Jonathan Roberts. 2015. 'Vaccination Persuasion Online: A Qualitative Study of Two Provaccine and Two Vaccine-Skeptical Websites'. *Journal of Medical Internet Research* 17 (5): e4153. <https://doi.org/10.2196/JMIR.4153>.

Green, Alex. 2017. 'Going Viral in the Online Anti-Vaccine Wars'. Wellcome Collection. <https://wellcomecollection.org/articles/Whf_BSkAACsAgwil>.

Greene, Jeremy A., Flurin Condrau, and Elizabeth Siegel Watkins. 2016. 'Therapeutic Revolutions: Pharmaceuticals and Social Change in the Twentieth Century'. *Therapeutic Revolutions*, November. <https://doi.org/10.7208/chicago/9780226390901.001.0001>.

Greenhough, Beth. 2012. 'Where Species Meet and Mingle: Endemic Human-Virus Relations, Embodied Communication and More-than-Human Agency at the Common Cold Unit 1946–90.' *Cultural Geographies* 19 (3): 281–301. <https://doi.org/10.1177/1474474011422029>.

Greenwood, Brian, Samba Sow, and Marie Pierre Preziosi. 2021. 'Defeating Meningitis by 2030 – an Ambitious Target'. *Transactions of the Royal Society of Tropical Medicine and Hygiene* 115 (10): 1099–101. <https://doi.org/10.1093/TRSTMH/TRAB133>.

Grignolio, Andrea. 2018. *Vaccines: are they Worth a Shot?* Cham: Springer.

Gross, M., & McGoey, L. (eds). 2015. *Routledge International Handbook of Ignorance Studies*. 1st ed. London: Routledge. <https://doi.org/10.4324/9781315867762>.

Guardian. 2020. 'UK Vaccine Trial Volunteer Says She Is "Doing Fine" after Online Death Rumours'. <https://www.theguardian.com/world/2020/apr/26/uk-coronavirus-vaccine-trial-subject-doing-fine-online-death-rumours-elisa-granato?CMP=fb_gu&utm_medium=Social&utm_source=Facebook>.

Hajer, Maarten A. 2009. *Authoritative Governance: Policy-Making in the Age of Mediatization*. Oxford: Oxford University Press.

Hajj Hussein, Inaya, Nour Chams, Sana Chams, Skye El Sayegh, Reina Badran, Mohamad Raad, Alice Gerges-Geagea, Angelo Leone, and Abdo Jurjus. 2015. 'Vaccines through Centuries: Major Cornerstones of Global Health'. *Frontiers in Public Health* 3 (November): 269. <https://doi.org/10.3389/fpubh.2015.00269>.

Hanney, Stephen R., Steven Wooding, Jon Sussex, and Jonathan Grant. 2020. 'From COVID-19 Research to Vaccine Application: Why Might It Take 17 Months Not 17 Years and What Are the Wider Lessons?' *Health Research Policy and Systems* 18 (1): 61. <https://doi.org/10.1186/s12961-020-00571-3>.

Hansen, Jane. 2013a. 'Grieving Parents Speak Out against Anti-Vaccination Extremists'. *Daily Telegraph*. <https://www.dailytelegraph.com.au/news/opinion/grieving-parents-speak-out-against-anti-vaccination-extremists/news-story/2b0a81b5b3f391f42903bfb52851d7df>.

Hansen, Jane. 2013b. 'No Jab, No Play Campaign Launched to Ban Unvaccinated Kids from Childcare Centres and Preschools'. *Daily Telegraph*. <https://www.dailytelegraph.com.au/news/national/no-jab-no-play-campaign-launched-to-ban-unvaccinated-kids-from-childcare-centres-and-preschools/news-story/7fc848cff24a95927c94cadc927f77b7>.

Harding, Emma, Philip Robinson, James Wilson, Sebastian J. Crutch, and Catherine J. Mummery. 2021. 'Injections of Hope: Supporting Participants in Clinical Trials'. *BMJ* 375 (December): e066851. <https://doi.org/10.1136/BMJ-2021-066851>.

Hart, Angie, Ceri Davies, Kim Aumann, Etienne Wenger, Kay Aranda, Becky Heaver, and David Wolff. 2013. 'Mobilising Knowledge in Community–University Partnerships: What Does a Community of Practice Approach Contribute?' *Contemporary Social Science* 8 (3): 278–91. <https://doi.org/10.1080/21582041.2013.767470>.

Harvey, Amanda M., Sharlynn Thompson, Andrew Lac, and Frederick L. Coolidge. 2019. 'Fear and Derision: A Quantitative Content Analysis of Provaccine and Antivaccine Internet Memes'. *Health Education and Behavior* 46 (6): 1012–23. <https://doi.org/10.1177/1090198119866886>.

Hausman, Bernice L. 2019. *Anti/Vax: Reframing the Vaccination Controversy*. Ithaca, NY: Cornell University Press.

Health Care Complaints Commission. 2014. 'Public Statement – Warning about the Australian Vaccination-Skeptics Network, Inc. ("AVN"), Formerly Known as Australian Vaccination Network Inc.' NSW Government Webpage. Health Care Complaints Commission. <http://www.hccc.nsw.gov.au/Hearings---decisions/Public-statements-and-warnings/Public-statement---warning-about-the-Australian-Vaccination-skeptics-Network--Inc---AVN----formerly-known-as-Australian-Vaccination-Network-Inc->.

Healy, Jack, and Michael Paulson. 2015. 'Vaccine Critics Turn Defensive Over Measles'. *New York Times*. <https://www.nytimes.com/2015/01/31/us/vaccine-critics-turn-defensive-over-measles.html>.

Herasimenka, Aliaksandr, Jonathan Bright, Aleksi Knuutila, and Philip N. Howard. 2022. 'Misinformation and Professional News on Largely Unmoderated Platforms: The Case of Telegram.' *Journal of Information Technology & Politics* 20:2. 198–212. https://www.tandfonline.com/doi/pdf/10.1080/19331681.2022.2076272>.

Hernandez, Adrian. 2020. 'Covid-19 Clinical Trial Pauses "Show the System Is Working"'. *STAT*. <https://www.statnews.com/2020/10/14/covid-19-clinical-trial-pauses-show-the-system-is-working/>.

Hijazi, Rana, Anat Gesser-Edelsburg, Paula Feder-Bubis, and Gustavo S. Mesch. 2022. 'Pro-Vaccination Groups Expressing Hesitant Attitudes: A Cross-Sectional Study about the Difference between Attitudes and Actual Behavior in Israel'. *Frontiers in Public Health* 10 (April): 1096. <https://www.ncbi.nlm.nih.gov/pmc/articles/PMC9092369/>.

Hill, Matilda, Samantha Vanderslott, Alla Volokha, and Andrew J Pollard. 2022. 'Addressing Vaccine Inequities among Ukrainian Refugees'. *Lancet Infectious Diseases* 22 (7): 935–6. <https://doi.org/10.1016/S1473-3099(22)00366-8>.

Hilleman, Maurice R. 2000. 'Vaccines in Historic Evolution and Perspective: A Narrative of Vaccine Discoveries'. *Vaccine* 18 (15): 1436–47. <https://doi.org/10.1016/S0264-410X(99)00434-X>.

Hindu. 2017. 'MR Vaccine Drive: A Call to Immunise One and All'. <https://www.thehindu.com/news/national/mr-vaccine-drive-unicef-reaches-out-to-islamic-civil-society-organisations/article17930240.ece>.

Hobson-West, Pru. 2007. '"Trusting Blindly Can Be the Biggest Risk of All": Organised Resistance to Childhood Vaccination in the UK'. *Sociology of Health & Illness* 29 (2): 198–215. <https://doi.org/10.1111/j.1467-9566.2007.00544.x>.

Hood, Gillian A., Tahseen A. Chowdhury, Christopher J. Griffiths, Rosie K. E. Hood, Christopher Mathews, and Graham A. Hitman. 2015. 'The Mela Study: Exploring Barriers to Diabetes Research in Black and Minority Ethnic Groups'. *Primary Health Care Research & Development* 16 (1): 53–60. <https://doi.org/10.1017/S1463423614000061>.

Hornsey, Matthew J., Martin Edwards, Josep Lobera, Celia Díaz-Catalán, and Fiona Kate Barlow. 2021. 'Resolving the Small-Pockets Problem Helps Clarify the Role of Education and Political Ideology in Shaping Vaccine Scepticism'. *British Journal of Psychology* 112 (4): 992–1011. <https://doi.org/10.1111/BJOP.12500>.

Howard, Jacqueline. 2017. 'Anti-vaccine Groups Blamed in Minnesota Measles Outbreak'. *CNN*. <https://edition.cnn.com/2017/05/08/health/measles-minnesota-somali-anti-vaccine-bn/index.html>.

Hughes, Michael J., Meseret G. Birhane, Layne Dorough, Jared L. Reynolds, Hayat Caidi, Kaitlin A. Tagg, Caroline M. Snyder, et al. 2021. 'Extensively Drug-Resistant Typhoid Fever in the United States'. *Open Forum Infectious Diseases* 8 (12). <https://doi.org/10.1093/ofid/ofab572>.

Hussain, Rashid S., Stephen T. McGarvey, Tabassam Shahab, and Lina M. Fruzzetti. 2012. 'Fatigue and Fear with Shifting Polio Eradication Strategies in India: A

Study of Social Resistance to Vaccination'. *PLoS ONE* 7 (9): e46274. <https://doi.org/10.1371/journal.pone.0046274>.

Hutchings, Matt, Andrew Truman, and Barrie Wilkinson. 2019. 'Antibiotics: Past, Present and Future'. *Current Opinion in Microbiology* 51 (October): 72–80. <https://doi.org/10.1016/J.MIB.2019.10.008>.

Im, Justin, Farhana Khanam, Faisal Ahmmed, Deok Ryun Kim, Sophie Kang, Birkneh Tilahun Tadesse, Fahima Chowdhury, et al. 2022. 'Prevention of Typhoid Fever by Existing Improvements in Household Water, Sanitation, and Hygiene, and the Use of the Vi Polysaccharide Typhoid Vaccine in Poor Urban Slums: Results from a Cluster-Randomized Trial'. *American Journal of Tropical Medicine and Hygiene* 106 (4): 1149–55. <https://doi.org/10.4269/AJTMH.21-1034>.

Irwin, Alan. 2006. 'The Politics of Talk: Coming to Terms with the 'New' scientific Governance'. *Social Studies of Science* 36 (2): 299–320.

Islam, Md Saiful, Abu Hena Mostofa Kamal, Alamgir Kabir, Dorothy L. Southern, Sazzad Hossain Khan, S. M. Murshid Hasan, Tonmoy Sarkar, et al. 2021. 'COVID-19 Vaccine Rumors and Conspiracy Theories: The Need for Cognitive Inoculation against Misinformation to Improve Vaccine Adherence'. *PLOS ONE* 16 (5): e0251605. <https://doi.org/10.1371/JOURNAL.PONE.0251605>.

Jackson, Cath, Joanne Yarwood, Vanessa Saliba, and Helen Bedford. 2017. 'UK Parents' Attitudes towards Meningococcal Group B (MenB) Vaccination: A Qualitative Analysis'. *BMJ Open* 7 (4): e012851. <https://doi.org/10.1136/BMJOPEN-2016-012851>.

Jacob John, T., and Valsan P. Verghese. 2011. 'Time to Re-think Measles Vaccination Schedule in India'. *Indian Journal of Medical Research* 134 (3): 256. <https://www.ncbi.nlm.nih.gov/pmc/articles/PMC3193705/>.

Jacobs, Charlotte. 2015. *Jonas Salk: A Life*. Oxford: Oxford University Press.

Jacobson, Robert M. 2010. 'Vaccination Refusal and Parental Education: Lessons Learnt and Future Challenges'. *Pediatric Health* 4 (3): 239–42. <https://doi.org/10.2217/phe.10.27>.

Jacobson, Robert M., and Lila J. Finney Rutten. 2019. 'Parent's Hesitance about HPV Vaccine: Using the CASE Approach to Address Their Concerns'. *Minnesota Medicine* 102: 24–27. <http://www.ncbi.nlm.nih.gov/pubmed/34531616>.

Jamka, Leslie P., Kenneth W. Simiyu, Adwoa D. Bentsi-Enchill, Aziza J. Mwisongo, Helen Matzger, Anthony A. Marfin, Andrew J. Pollard, and Kathleen M. Neuzil. 2019. 'Accelerating Typhoid Conjugate Vaccine Introduction: What Can Be Learned from Prior New Vaccine Introduction Initiatives?' *Clinical Infectious Diseases* 68 (suppl. 2): S171–76. <https://doi.org/10.1093/CID/CIY1118>.

Jamrozik, Euzebiusz, and Michael J. Selgelid. 2021. 'History of Human Challenge Studies'. *SpringerBriefs in Ethics*, 9–23. <https://doi.org/10.1007/978-3-030-41480-1_2>.

Jamrozik, Euzebiusz, Katherine Littler, Susan Bull, Claudia Emerson, Gagandeep Kang, Melissa Kapulu, Elena Rey, et al. 2021. 'Key Criteria for the Ethical Acceptability of COVID-19 Human Challenge Studies: Report of a WHO Working Group'. *Vaccine* 39 (4): 633–40. <https://doi.org/10.1016/J.VACCINE.2020.10.075>.

Jané, Mireia, Maria José Vidal, Neus Camps, Magda Campins, Ana Martínez, Joan Balcells, Maria Teresa Martin-Gomez, et al. 2018. 'A Case of Respiratory Toxigenic Diphtheria: Contact Tracing Results and Considerations Following a 30-Year Disease-Free Interval, Catalonia, Spain, 2015'. *Eurosurveillance* 23 (13): 17–00183. <https://pubmed.ncbi.nlm.nih.gov/29616610/>.

Jane, Sinduja. 2017. 'Tamil Nadu Government to Take on Trolls against Measles-Rubella Vaccine Drive'. *New Indian Express*. <https://www.newindianexpress.com/states/tamil-nadu/2017/jan/31/tamil-nadu-government-to-take-on-trolls-against-measles-rubella-vaccine-drive-1565378.html>.

Jao, Irene, Vicki Marsh, Primus Che Chi, Melissa Kapulu, Mainga Hamaluba, Sassy Molyneux, Philip Bejon, and Dorcas Kamuya. 2020. 'Deliberately Infecting Healthy Volunteers with Malaria Parasites: Perceptions and Experiences of Participants and Other Stakeholders in a Kenyan-Based Malaria Infection Study'. *Bioethics* 34 (8): 819–32. <https://doi.org/10.1111/BIOE.12781>.

Jarrett, Caitlin, Rose Wilson, Maureen O'Leary, Elisabeth Eckersberger, Heidi J. Larson, Juhani Eskola, Xiaofeng Liang, et al. 2015. 'Strategies for Addressing Vaccine Hesitancy – a Systematic Review'. *Vaccine* 33 (34): 4180–90. <https://doi.org/10.1016/J.VACCINE.2015.04.040>.

Jayarajan, Nayana. 2020. 'Religious Communities & Vaccines: Lessons from Polio Campaign'. *New Indian Express*. <https://www.newindianexpress.com/opinions/2020/sep/21/religious-communities-vaccines-lessons-from-polio-campaign-2199712.html>.

Jeffery, Patricia, and Roger Jeffery. 2011. 'Underserved and Overdosed? Muslims and the Pulse Polio Initiative in Rural North India'. *Contemporary South Asia* 19 (2): 117–35. <https://doi.org/10.1080/09584935.2010.537744>.

Johnston, Robert D. 2004. *The Politics of Healing: Histories of Alternative Medicine in Twentieth-Century North America*. New York: Routledge.

Kadambari, Seilesh, and Samantha Vanderslott. 2021. 'Lessons about COVID-19 Vaccine Hesitancy among Minority Ethnic People in the UK'. *Lancet Infectious Diseases* 21 (9): 1204–6. <https://doi.org/10.1016/S1473-3099(21)00404-7>.

Kahan, Dan M. 2014. 'Vaccine Risk Perceptions and Ad Hoc Risk Communication: An Empirical Assessment'. *SSRN Electronic Journal*, January. <https://doi.org/10.2139/SSRN.2386034>.

Kalra, Suprita P., Nardeep Naithani, Shivram R. Mehta, and Ajay Jagannath Swamy. 2003. 'Current Trends in the Management of Typhoid Fever'. *Medical Journal, Armed Forces India* 59 (2): 130. <https://doi.org/10.1016/S0377-1237(03)80060-6>.

Kasstan, Ben. 2019. *Making Bodies Kosher: The Politics of Reproduction among Haredi Jews in England*. New York: Berghahn.

Kasstan, Ben. 2021. '"If a Rabbi Did Say 'You Have to Vaccinate', We Wouldn't": Unveiling the Secular Logics of Religious Exemption and Opposition to Vaccination'. *Social Science and Medicine* 280 (July): 114052. <https://doi.org/10.1016/j.socscimed.2021.114052>.

Kasstan, Ben, Sandra Mounier-Jack, Louise Letley, Katherine M. Gaskell, Chrissy H. Roberts, Neil R.H. Stone, Sham Lal, Rosalind M. Eggo, Michael Marks, and Tracey Chantler. 2022. 'Localising Vaccination Services: Qualitative Insights on Public Health and Minority Group Collaborations to Co-Deliver Coronavirus Vaccines'. *Vaccine* 40 (14): 2226–32. <https://doi.org/10.1016/J.VACCINE.2022.02.056>.

Kata, Anna. 2012. 'Anti-vaccine activists, Web 2.0, and the postmodern paradigm—an overview of tactics and tropes used online by the anti-vaccination movement'. *Vaccine*, 30 (25): 3778–3789. <https://doi.org/10.1016/j.vaccine.2011.11.112>

Faasse, Kate, Casey J. Chatman, and Leslie R. Martin. 2016. 'A Comparison of Language Use in Pro- and Anti-vaccination Comments in Response to a High Profile Facebook Post'. *Vaccine* 34 (47): 5808–14. <https://doi.org/10.1016/J.VACCINE.2016.09.029>.

O'Neill, Katie. 2020. 'Oxford Coronavirus Vaccine Trial on Hold after Suspected Adverse Reaction'. *Telegraph*. <https://www.telegraph.co.uk/news/2020/09/08/oxford-coronavirus-vaccine-trial-hold-suspected-adverse-reaction/>.

Kaul, Rhythma. 2017. 'Second Phase of Measles-Rubella Vaccination Drive Launched in Eight States, UTs'. *Hindustan Times*. <https://www.hindustantimes.com/health/second-phase-of-measles-rubella-vaccination-drive-launched-in-eight-states-uts/story-poDkt10IQpOfoFohmPD3ZL.html>.

Keja, Ko, Carole Chan, Gregory Hayden, and Ralph H. Henderson. 1988. 'Expanded Programme on Immunization. *World Health Statistics Quarterly* 41(2): 59–63. <https://pubmed.ncbi.nlm.nih.gov/3176515/>.

Kelland, Kate, and Pavel Polityuk. 2019. 'Measles and Mistrust in Ukraine Weaken World's Defenses'. *Reuters*. <https://www.reuters.com/article/idUSKBN1XE15S/>.

Kennedy, David A., and Andrew F. Read. 2018. 'Why the Evolution of Vaccine Resistance Is Less of a Concern than the Evolution of Drug Resistance'. *Proceedings of the National Academy of Sciences of the United States of America* 115 (51): 12878. <https://doi.org/10.1073/PNAS.1717159115>.

Kennedy, Jonathan, and Domna Michailidou. 2015. 'Militant Islamism and Vaccine Skepticism'. *Project Syndicate*. <https://www.project-syndicate.org/commentary/islamist-polio-vaccination-opposition-by-jonathan-kennedy-and-domna-michailidou-2015-10#comments>.

Kenneth, David F., Rachael Kiple, Graham Rockwell, David Frey, and Alicia Browne. 1993. 'The Cambridge World History of Human Disease'. *Cambridge World History of Human Disease*, January. <https://doi.org/10.1017/CHOL9780521332866>.

Khatami, Ameneh, and Andrew J. Pollard. 2014. 'The Epidemiology of Meningococcal Disease and the Impact of Vaccines'. *Expert Review Vaccines* 9 (3): 285–98. <https://doi.org/10.1586/ERV.10.3>.

Khimm, Suzy. 2010. 'Did the Anti-vaccine Movement Help Create a Whooping Cough Epidemic?' *Mother Jones*. <http://www.motherjones.com/kevin-drum/2010/06/vaccines-california-whooping-cough-epidemic/>.

Kirby, Jane. 2022. '"I'm Just an Ordinary Bloke": Man Recalls Son as He Continues Meningitis Fight'. *The Independent*. 2022. <https://www.independent.co.uk/news/uk/spencer-mbe-bristol-calpol-b2065337.html>.

Kirchhelle, Claas, and Samantha Vanderslott. 2019. 'Decades Neglecting an Ancient Disease Has Triggered a Health Emergency around the World'. *Conversation*. <https://theconversation.com/decades-neglecting-an-ancient-disease-has-triggered-a-health-emergency-around-the-world-121282>.

Kirchhelle, Claas, and Samantha Vanderslott. 2021. 'Editorial: The Need for Harmonised International Guidelines Ahead of COVID-19 Human Infection Studies'. *Public Health Reviews* (January): 2. <https://doi.org/10.3389/PHRS.2021.1603962>.

Kirchhelle, Claas, Zoe Anne Dyson, and Gordon Dougan. 2019. 'A Biohistorical Perspective of Typhoid and Antimicrobial Resistance'. *Clinical Infectious Diseases* 69 (suppl. 5): S388–94. <https://doi.org/10.1093/cid/ciz556>.

Kirchhelle, Claas, Paul Atkinson, Alex Broom, Komatra Chuengsatiansup, Jorge Pinto Ferreira, Nicolas Fortané, Isabel Frost, et al. 2020. 'Setting the Standard: Multidisciplinary Hallmarks for Structural, Equitable and Tracked Antibiotic Policy'. *BMJ Global Health* 5 (9): e003091. <https://doi.org/10.1136/BMJGH-2020-003091>.

Knepper, Todd C., and Howard L. McLeod. 2018. 'When Will Clinical Trials Finally Reflect Diversity? Comment'. *Nature*. <https://doi.org/10.1038/d41586-018-05049-5>.

Kuran, Timur. 1995. *Private Truths, Public Lies: The Social Consequences of Preference Falsification*. Cambridge: Harvard University Press.

Kuru, Ozan, Man pui Sally Chan, Hang Lu, Dominik Andrzej Stecula, Kathleen Hall Jamieson, and Dolores Albarracín. 2022. 'Religious Affiliation and Philosophical and Moral Beliefs about Vaccines: A Longitudinal Study'. *Journal of Health Psychology* 27 (13): 3059–81. <https://www.ncbi.nlm.nih.gov/pmc/articles/PMC9580036/>.

Kyriakidis, Nikolaos C., Andrés López-Cortés, Eduardo Vásconez González, Alejandra Barreto Grimaldos, and Esteban Ortiz Prado. 2021. 'SARS-CoV-2 Vaccines Strategies: A Comprehensive Review of Phase 3 Candidates'. *Npj Vaccines* 6 (1): 1–17. <https://doi.org/10.1038/s41541-021-00292-w>.

Ladhani, Shamez N., Nick Andrews, Sydel R. Parikh, Helen Campbell, Joanne White, Michael Edelstein, Xilian Bai, Jay Lucidarme, Ray Borrow, and Mary E. Ramsay. 2020. 'Vaccination of Infants with Meningococcal Group B Vaccine (4CMenB) in England'. *New England Journal of Medicine* 382 (4): 309–17. <https://www.nejm.org/doi/full/10.1056/NEJMoa1901229>.

Laforce, F. Marc, Mamoudou Djingarey, Simonetta Viviani, and Marie Pierre Preziosi. 2017. 'Lessons from the Meningitis Vaccine Project'. *Viral Immunology* 31 (2): 109–13. <https://doi.org/10.1089/VIM.2017.0120>.

Lahariya, Chandrakant. 2014. 'A Brief History of Vaccines and Vaccination in India'. *Indian Journal of Medical Research* 139 (4): 491–511. <http://www.ncbi.nlm.nih.gov/pubmed/24927336>.

Lambkin-Williams, Rob, Nicolas Noulin, Alex Mann, Andrew Catchpole, and Anthony S. Gilbert. 2018. 'The Human Viral Challenge Model: Accelerating the Evaluation of Respiratory Antivirals, Vaccines and Novel Diagnostics'. *Respiratory Research* 19 (1): 1–15. <https://doi.org/10.1186/S12931-018-0784-1>.

Lancet, The Editors of the. 2010. 'Retraction-Ileal-Lymphoid-Nodular Hyperplasia, Non-Specific Colitis, and Pervasive Developmental Disorder in Children'. *Lancet* 375 (9713): 445. <https://doi.org/10.1016/S0140-6736(10)60175-4>.

Larson, Heidi J. 2018. 'The Biggest Pandemic Risk? Viral Misinformation'. *Nature* 562: 7727, October.

Larson, Heidi J., Rose Wilson, Sharon Hanley, Astrid Parys, and Pauline Paterson. 2014. 'Tracking the Global Spread of Vaccine Sentiments: The Global Response to Japan's Suspension of Its HPV Vaccine Recommendation'. *Human Vaccines & Immunotherapeutics* 10 (9): 2543. <https://doi.org/10.4161/21645515.2014.969618>.

Larson, Heidi J., Alexandre de Figueiredo, Zhao Xiahong, William S. Schulz, Pierre Verger, Iain G. Johnston, Alex R. Cook, and Nick S. Jones. 2016a. 'The State of Vaccine Confidence 2016: Global Insights through a 67-Country

Survey'. *EBioMedicine* 12 (October): 295–301. <https://doi.org/10.1016/j.ebiom.2016.08.042>.

Leach, Melissa, and James Fairhead. 2007. *Vaccine Anxieties: Global Science, Child Health and Society*. London: Earthscan.

Leask, Julie, and Margie Danchin. 2017. 'Imposing Penalties for Vaccine Rejection Requires Strong Scrutiny'. *Journal of Paediatrics and Child Health* 53 (5): 439–44. <https://doi.org/10.1111/jpc.13472>.

Leavitt, Judith Walzer. 1996. *Typhoid Mary: Captive to the Public's Health*. Boston: Beacon Press. <https://quod.lib.umich.edu/cgi/t/text/text-idx?c=acls;cc=acls;view=toc;idno=heb02042.0001.001>.

Lee, Sun Kyong, Juhyung Sun, Seulki Jang, and Shane Connelly. 2022. 'Misinformation of COVID-19 Vaccines and Vaccine Hesitancy'. *Scientific Reports* 12 (1): 1–11. <https://doi.org/10.1038/s41598-022-17430-6>.

Leston-Bandeira, Cristina. 2019. 'Parliamentary Petitions and Public Engagement: An Empirical Analysis of the Role of e-Petitions'. *Policy & Politics* 47 (3): 415–36. <https://doi.org/10.1332/030557319X15579230420117>.

Lipsitch, Marc, and George R. Siber. 2016. 'How Can Vaccines Contribute to Solving the Antimicrobial Resistance Problem?' *MBio* 7 (3): 1–8. <https://doi.org/10.1128/MBIO.00428-16>.

Loomba, S., A. de Figueiredo, S. J. Piatek, et al. 2021. 'Measuring the Impact of COVID-19 Vaccine Misinformation on Vaccination Intent in the UK and USA'. *Nature Human Behaviour* 5: 337–348. <https://doi.org/10.1038/s41562-021-01056-1>.

Loxton, Daniel. n.d. 'Modern Skepticism's Unique Mandate'. Skepticblog. Accessed 7 August 2017. <http://www.skepticblog.org/2013/05/13/modern-skepticisms-unique-mandate/>.

Lutkenhaus, Roel O., Jeroen Jansz, and Martine P. A. Bouman. 2019. 'Mapping the Dutch Vaccination Debate on Twitter: Identifying Communities, Narratives, and Interactions'. *Vaccine: X* 1 (April): 100019. <https://doi.org/10.1016/J.JVACX.2019.100019>.

Lynch, Holly Fernandez, Emily A. Largent, Steven Joffe, and Angela M. DeMichele. 2018. 'Protecting Clinical Trial Participants and Study Integrity in the Age of Social Media.' *Cancer* 124 (24): 4610–17. <https://doi.org/10.1002/CNCR.31748>.

MacDonald, Noni E., Juhani Eskola, Xiaofeng Liang, Mohuya Chaudhuri, Eve Dubé, Bruce Gellin, Susan Goldstein, et al. 2015. 'Vaccine Hesitancy: Definition, Scope and Determinants'. *Vaccine* 33 (34): 4161–4. <https://doi.org/10.1016/J.VACCINE.2015.04.036>.

Mach, Katharine J., Raúl Salas Reyes, Brian Pentz, Jennifer Taylor, Clarissa A. Costa, Sandip G. Cruz, Kerronia E. Thomas, et al. 2021. 'News Media

Coverage of COVID-19 Public Health and Policy Information'. *Humanities and Social Sciences Communications* 8 (1): 1–11. <https://doi.org/10.1057/s41599-021-00900-z>.

Maciuszek, Józef, Mateusz Polak, Katarzyna Stasiuk, and Dariusz Doliński. 2021. 'Active Pro-vaccine and Anti-vaccine Groups: Their Group Identities and Attitudes toward Science'. *PLOS ONE* 16 (12): e0261648. <https://doi.org/10.1371/JOURNAL.PONE.0261648>.

Mackey, Katherine, Chelsea K. Ayers, Karli K. Kondo, Somnath Saha, Shailesh M. Advani, Sarah Young, Hunter Spencer, et al. 2021. 'Racial and Ethnic Disparities in COVID-19-Related Infections, Hospitalizations, and Deaths : A Systematic Review'. *Annals of Internal Medicine* 174 (3): 362–73. <https://doi.org/10.7326/M20-6306>.

MacLennan, Jenny M., Charlene M. C. Rodrigues, Holly B. Bratcher, Aiswarya Lekshmi, Adam Finn, Jenny Oliver, Mandy Wootton, et al. 2021. 'Meningococcal Carriage in Periods of High and Low Invasive Meningococcal Disease Incidence in the UK: Comparison of UKMenCar1–4 Cross-Sectional Survey Results'. *Lancet Infectious Diseases* 21 (5): 677. <https://doi.org/10.1016/S1473-3099(20)30842-2>.

Mahase, Elisabeth. 2020. Covid-19: UK Starts Social Distancing After New Model Points to 260 000 Potential Deaths. *BMJ* 368: m1089.

Mahase, Elisabeth. 2021. 'Covid-19: Where Are We on Vaccines and Variants?' *BMJ* 372 (March): n597. <https://doi.org/10.1136/bmj.n597>.

Majumder, Maimuna S., and Kenneth D. Mandl. 2020. 'Early in the Epidemic: Impact of Preprints on Global Discourse about COVID-19 Transmissibility'. *Lancet Global Health* 8 (5): e627. <https://doi.org/10.1016/S2214-109X(20)30113-3>.

Marsh, Abigail A., Monica Magalhaes, Matthew Peeler, Sophie M. Rose, Thomas C. Darton, Nir Eyal, Josh Morrison, Seema K. Shah, and Virginia Schmit. 2022. 'Characterizing Altruistic Motivation in Potential Volunteers for SARS-CoV-2 Challenge Trials'. *PLOS ONE* 17 (11): e0275823. <https://doi.org/10.1371/JOURNAL.PONE.0275823>.

Martin, Brian. 2016. 'An Experience with Vaccination Gatekeepers'. *Social Epistemology Review and Reply Collective* 5 (10): 27–33.

Martin, Sam, and Samantha Vanderslott. 2021. '"Any Idea How Fast 'It's Just a Mask!' Can Turn into 'It's Just a Vaccine!'": From Mask Mandates to Vaccine Mandates during the COVID-19 Pandemic'. *Vaccine*, October. <https://doi.org/10.1016/J.VACCINE.2021.10.031>.

Masignani, Vega, Mariagrazia Pizza, and Richard Moxon. 2019. 'The Development of a Vaccine against Meningococcus B Using Reverse Vaccinology'. *Frontiers in Immunology* 10 (Mar): 751. <https://doi.org/10.3389/fimmu.2019.00751>.

McBrien, Jacqueline, John Murphy, Denis Gill, Mary Cronin, Catherine O'Donovan, and Mary T. Cafferkey. 2003. 'Measles Outbreak in Dublin, 2000'. *Pediatric Infectious Disease Journal* 22 (7): 580–4. <https://doi.org/10.1097/01.INF.0000073059.57867.36>.

McCarthy, John D., and Mayer N. Zald. 1977. 'Resource Mobilization and Social Movements: A Partial Theory'. *American Journal of Sociology* 82: 1212–1241. <https://doi.org/10.1086/226464>.

McInerney, Fran. 2000. 'Requested Death: A New Social Movement'. *Social Science & Medicine* 50 (1): 137–54. <https://doi.org/10.1016/S0277-936(99)00273-7>.

McIntyre, Peter B., Katherine L. O'Brien, Brian Greenwood, and Diederik Van De Beek. 2012. 'Effect of Vaccines on Bacterial Meningitis Worldwide'. *Lancet* 380 (9854): 1703–11. <https://doi.org/10.1016/S0140-6736(12)61187-8>.

McNeil, Donald. G. 2009. 'Book Is Rallying Resistance to the Antivaccine Crusade'. *New York Times*. <http://www.nytimes.com/2009/01/13/health/13auti.html>.

Meiring, James E., Alberto Giubilini, Julian Savulescu, Virginia E. Pitzer, and Andrew J. Pollard. 2019. 'Generating the Evidence for Typhoid Vaccine Introduction: Considerations for Global Disease Burden Estimates and Vaccine Testing Through Human Challenge'. *Clinical Infectious Diseases* 69 (suppl. 5): S402–7. <https://doi.org/10.1093/CID/CIZ630>.

Meningitis Now. n.d. 'Meningitis B Campaign Timeline'. Accessed 19 August 2022. <https://www.meningitisnow.org/support-us/news-centre/public-affairs/campaigns/beat-it-now/campaign-timeline/>.

Merton, Robert K. 1942. 'The Normative Structure of Science'. The sociology of science: Theoretical and empirical investigations, 267–78. <https://www.panarchy.org/merton/science.html>.

Meryl Dorey. n.d. 'Why I Did What I Did – Why I Do What I Do by Meryl Dorey'. Whale.To. Accessed 16 July 2017. <http://www.whale.to/vaccine/dorey.html>.

Miles, David. 2023. *How Vaccines Work : The Science and History behind Every Question You've Wanted To Ask*. London: Piatkus.

Milken Institute School of Public Health. 2015. 'Q&A with Tara Haelle: Time to Overhaul How We Talk about Health'. MISPH Blog. <https://onlinepublichealth.gwu.edu/resources/national-immunization-awareness-month-2015-vaccination/>.

Miller, Sara G., and Erika Edwards. 2020. 'Oxford Vaccine Trial on Hold Because of Potential Safety Issue.' *NBC*. <https://www.nbcnews.com/health/health-news/oxford-vaccine-trial-hold-due-safety-issue-n1239581>.

Mills, Edward, Curtis Cooper, Gordon Guyatt, Amy Gilchrist, Beth Rachlis, Chris Sulway, and Kumanan Wilson. 2004. 'Barriers to Participating in an HIV

Vaccine Trial: A Systematic Review'. *AIDS* 18 (17): 2235–42. <https://doi.org/10.1097/00002030-200411190-00003>.

Mohan, Vadrevu Krishna, Vineeth Varanasi, Anit Singh, Marcela F. Pasetti, Myron M. Levine, Ramasamy Venkatesan, and Krishna M. Ella. 2015. 'Safety and Immunogenicity of a Vi Polysaccharide-Tetanus Toxoid Conjugate Vaccine (Typbar-TCV) in Healthy Infants, Children, and Adults in Typhoid Endemic Areas: A Multicenter, 2-Cohort, Open-Label, Double-Blind, Randomized Controlled Phase 3 Study'. *Clinical Infectious Diseases* 61 (3): 393–402. <https://doi.org/10.1093/CID/CIV295>.

Mohr, Kathrin I. 2016. 'History of Antibiotics Research'. *Current Topics in Microbiology and Immunology* 398 (December): 237–72. <https://pubmed.ncbi.nlm.nih.gov/27738915/>.

Moore, Ramey, Rachel S. Purvis, Don E. Willis, Kyle C. Worley, Devonte Hervey, Sharon Reece, Aimee Yeates, and Pearl A. McElfish. 2022. 'The Vaccine Hesitancy Continuum among Hesitant Adopters of the COVID-19 Vaccine'. *Clinical and Translational Science* 15 (12): 2844–57. <https://doi.org/10.1111/CTS.13385>.

Moore, Thomas. 2020. 'COVID-19: The Story of Oxford's Coronavirus Vaccine That Could Save Britain'. *Sky News*. <https://news.sky.com/story/covid-19-the-story-of-oxfords-coronavirus-vaccine-that-could-save-britain-12139898>.

Moskalenko, S., and C. McCauley. 2009. 'Measuring political mobilization: The distinction between activism and radicalism'. *Terrorism and Political Violence* 21 (2): 239–260.

Mouw, Ted, and Michael E. Sobel. 2015. 'Culture Wars and Opinion Polarization: The Case of Abortion'. *American Journal of Sociology* 10 (4): 913–43. <https://doi.org/10.1086/320294>.

Moxon, Richard. 2021. 'Brain Fever: How Vaccines Prevent Meningitis and Other Killer Diseases'. *Brain Fever: How Vaccines Prevent Meningitis and Other Killer Diseases*, London: World Scientific Europe Ltd. 1–264. <https://doi.org/10.1142/q0291>.

Murch, Simon H., Andrew Anthony, David H. Casson, Mohsin Malik, Mark Berelowitz, Amar P. Dhillon, Michael A. Thomson, Alan Valentine, Susan E. Davies, and John A. Walker-Smith. 2004. 'Retraction of an Interpretation'. *Lancet* 363 (9411): 750. <https://doi.org/10.1016/S0140-6736(04)15715-2>.

Murphy, Margi. 2019. 'Dr Google Will See You Now: Search Giant Wants to Cash in on Your Medical Queries'. *Telegraph*. <https://www.telegraph.co.uk/technology/2019/03/10/google-sifting-one-billion-health-questions-day/>.

Mwale, Shadreck. 2017. *Healthy Volunteers in Commercial Clinical Drug Trials: When Human Beings Become Guinea Pigs*, Cham: Springer. 1–150. <https://link.springer.com/book/10.1007/978-3-319-59214-5>.

Mwale, Shadreck. 2020. '"Becoming-With" a Repeat Healthy Volunteer: Managing and Negotiating Trust among Repeat Healthy Volunteers in Commercial Clinical Drug Trials'. *Social Science & Medicine* 245 (January): 112670. <https://doi.org/10.1016/J.SOCSCIMED.2019.112670>.

Nair, Navin. 2017. '"Won't Take Modi-RSS Vaccine": Myths, Quacks Derail Malappuram Vaccination Drive Putting Lakhs of Children at Risk'. *Firstpost*. December 1. <https://www.firstpost.com/india/wont-take-modi-rss-vaccine-myths-quacks-derail-malappuram-vaccination-drive-putting-lakhs-of-children-at-risk-4236543.html>.

National Conference of State Legislatures. n.d. 'States with Religious and Philosophical Exemptions from School Immunization Requirements'. Accessed 2 April 2023. <https://www.ncsl.org/health/states-with-religious-and-philosophical-exemptions-from-school-immunization-requirements>.

NHS. n.d. 'MenACWY Vaccine'. Accessed 31 July 2022. <https://www.nhs.uk/conditions/vaccinations/men-acwy-vaccine/?>

Nichter, Mark. 1995. 'Vaccinations in the Third World: A Consideration of Community Demand'. *Social Science & Medicine* 41 (5): 617–32. <https://doi.org/10.1016/0277-9536(95)00034-5>.

Ophir, Yotam, Nathan Walter, Dror Walter, Raphaela M. Velho, Ayse D. Lokmanoglu, Meredith L. Pruden, and Emily A. Andrews. 2022. 'Vaccine Hesitancy under the Magnifying Glass: A Systematic Review of the Uses and Misuses of an Increasingly-Popular Construct'. *Health Communication*, March, 1–15. <https://doi.org/10.1080/10410236.2022.2054102>.

Orenstein, Walter A., and Alan R. Hinman. 1999. 'The Immunization System in the United States – the Role of School Immunization Laws'. *Vaccine* 17 (October): S19–24. <https://doi.org/10.1016/S0264-410X(99)00290-X>.

PA Media. 2020. 'UK Vaccine Trial Volunteer Says She Is "Doing Fine" after Online Death Rumours'. *Guardian*. 26 April. <https://www.theguardian.com/world/2020/apr/26/uk-coronavirus-vaccine-trial-subject-doing-fine-online-death-rumours-elisa-granato>.

Palacios, Ricardo, and Seema K. Shah. 2019. 'When Could Human Challenge Trials Be Deployed to Combat Emerging Infectious Diseases? Lessons from the Case of a Zika Virus Human Challenge Trial'. *Trials* 20 (suppl. 2): 1–8. <https://doi.org/10.1186/S13063-019-3843-0>.

Parikh, Sydel R., Helen Campbell, Julie A. Bettinger, Lee H. Harrison, Helen S. Marshall, Federico Martinon-Torres, Marco Aurelio Safadi, et al. 2020. 'The Everchanging Epidemiology of Meningococcal Disease Worldwide and the Potential for Prevention through Vaccination'. *Journal of Infection* 81 (4): 483–98. <https://doi.org/10.1016/J.JINF.2020.05.079>.

PATH. 2023. 'Multivalent Meningococcal Meningitis Vaccine from Serum Institute of India Achieves WHO Prequalification'. <https://www.path.org/media-center/multivalent-meningococcal-meningitis-vaccine-from-serum-institute-of-india-achieves-who-prequalification/>.

Patrick-Smith, Maia, Samantha Vanderslott, Katherine R. W. Emary, Susanne H. Hodgson, Tonia Thomas, Arabella S.V. Stuart. Andrew J. Pollard et al. 2024. 'Roles and Responsibilities of Participants, Researchers, and the Media in the Communication of Vaccine Trials: Experience from the United Kingdom's First Covid-19 Vaccine Trial'. *Vaccine*. 2024 Oct 1;42(26):126391. <https://doi:10.1016/j.vaccine.2024.126391.

Pepperrell Toby, F. Rodgers, P. Tandon, K. Sarsfield, M. Pugh-Jones, T. Rashid, and S. Keestra. 2021. 'Making a COVID-19 Vaccine That Works for Everyone: Ensuring Equity and Inclusivity in Clinical Trials'. *Global Health Action* 14 (1):1892309. <https://doi.org/10.1080/16549716.2021.1892309>.

Peretti-Watel, P., H. J. Larson, J. K. Ward, W. S. Schulz, P. Verger. 2015. 'Vaccine hesitancy: clarifying a theoretical framework for an ambiguous notion'. *PLoS Curr* 25: 7. <https://doi.org/10.1371/currents.outbreaks.6844c80ff9f5b273f34c91f71b7fc289>.

Pfizer. 2020. 'Pfizer and BioNTech Announce Vaccine Candidate Against Covid-19 Achieved Success in First Interim Analysis from Phase 3 Study'. <https://www.pfizer.com/news/press-release/press-release-detail/pfizer-and-biontech-announce-vaccine-candidate-against>.

PHE. 2015. 'Infection Report Invasive Meningococcal Disease (Laboratory Reports in England): 2014/2015 Annual Data by Epidemiological Year'. < https://assets.publishing.service.gov.uk/media/5a809409e5274a2e87dba9cb/hpr3815_imd-crrctd.pdf >.

Poland, Gregory A., Robert M. Jacobson, and Inna G. Ovsyannikova. 2009. 'Trends Affecting the Future of Vaccine Development and Delivery: The Role of Demographics, Regulatory Science, the Anti-Vaccine Movement, and Vaccinomics'. *Vaccine* 27 (25–26): 3240–44. <https://doi.org/10.1016/j.vaccine.2009.01.069>.

Porter, Dorothy, and Roy Porter. 1988. 'The Politics of Prevention: Anti-vaccinationism and Public Health in Nineteenth-Century England'. *Medical History* 32 (3): 231–52. <https://doi.org/10.1017/S0025727300048225>.

Prieto Curiel, Rafael, and Humberto González Ramírez. 2021. 'Vaccination Strategies against COVID-19 and the Diffusion of Anti-vaccination Views'. *Scientific Reports* 11 (1): 1–13. <https://doi.org/10.1038/s41598-021-85555-1>.

Qamar, Farah Naz, Rabab Batool, Sonia Qureshi, Miqdad Ali, Tahira Sadaf, Junaid Mehmood, Khalid Iqbal, Akram Sultan, Noah Duff, and Mohammad Tahir Yousafzai. 2020. 'Strategies to Improve Coverage of Typhoid Conjugate

Vaccine (TCV) Immunization Campaign in Karachi, Pakistan'. *Vaccines* 8 (4): 1–12. <https://doi.org/10.3390/VACCINES8040697>.

Raison, Stephanie. 2017. 'WhatsApp-Ening in India's Measles-Rubella Vaccine Campaign?' UNICEF Connect. <https://blogs.unicef.org/blog/whatsapp-ening-india-measles-rubella-campaign/>.

Rajan, Kaushik Sunder. 2005. 'Subjects of Speculation: Emergent Life Sciences and Market Logics in the United States and India'. *American Anthropologist* 107 (1): 19–30. <https://doi.org/10.1525/AA.2005.107.1.019>.

Rajan, Kaushik Sunder. 2017. *Pharmocracy: Value, Politics, and Knowledge in Global Biomedicine*. New York: Duke University Press. <https://doi.org/10.1515/9780822373285>.

Rana, Muhammad Suleman, Rana Jawad Asghar, Muhammad Usman, Aamer Ikram, Muhammad Salman, Massab Umair, Syed Sohail Zahoor Zaidi, Muhammad Anas, and Nadeem Ullah. 2022. 'The Resurgence of Wild Poliovirus in Pakistan and Afghanistan: A New Setback for Polio Eradication'. *Journal of Infection* 85 (3): 334–63. <https://doi.org/10.1016/J.JINF.2022.05.038>.

Ranji, Usha, and Alina Salganicoff. 2014. 'Data Note: Balancing on Shaky Ground: Women, Work and Family Health. The Kaiser Family Foundation. <http://www.kff.org/private-insurance/issue-brief/data-note-balancing-on-shaky-ground-women-work-and-family-health/>.

Rao, Menaka, and Vinita Govindarajan. 2017. 'WhatsApp Rumours about Vaccinations Hamper India's Drive to Halt Measles and Rubella'. *Scroll.In*. February 24. <https://scroll.in/pulse/830129/rumours-about-measles-rubella-vaccine-hit-coverage>.

Raymond, Meriel, Malick M. Gibani, Nicholas P. J. Day, and Phaik Yeong Cheah. 2019. 'Typhoidal Salmonella Human Challenge Studies: Ethical and Practical Challenges and Considerations for Low-Resource Settings'. *Trials* 20 (2): 1–7. <https://doi.org/10.1186/s13063-019-3844-z>.

Recio-Román, Almudena, Manuel Recio-Menéndez, and María Victoría Román-González. 2021. 'Vaccine Hesitancy and Political Populism: An Invariant Cross-European Perspective'. *International Journal of Environmental Research and Public Health* 18 (24): 1–20. <https://doi.org/10.3390/IJERPH182412953>.

Reuters. 2019. 'Facebook's WhatsApp Limits Users to Five Text Forwards to Curb Rumors'. 21 January. <https://www.reuters.com/article/facebook-whatsapp/facebooks-whatsapp-limits-text-forwards-to-5-recipients-to-curb-rumours-idUSL1N1ZL04B/>.

Reverby, Susan M. 2012. 'Ethical Failures and History Lessons: The U.S. Public Health Service Research Studies in Tuskegee and Guatemala'. *Public Health Reviews* 34 (1): 1–18. <https://doi.org/10.1007/BF03391665>.

Riedel, Stefan. 2005. 'Edward Jenner and the History of Smallpox and Vaccination'. *Proceedings* 18 (1): 21. <https://doi.org/10.1080/08998280.2005.11928028>.

Riesman, David. 1936. 'Deceased Diseases'. *Annals of Medical History* 8 (2): 160. <https://www.ncbi.nlm.nih.gov/pmc/articles/PMC7939838/>.

Ritzer, George. 2016. *Essentials of Sociology*. Los Angeles, CA: SAGE Publications.

Robinson, Steve, and Martha Priedeman Skiles. 2008. 'Development of a Measure of Vaccine Hesitancy'. <https://cdc.confex.com/cdc/nic2008/techprogram/P15811.HTM>

Rodríguez-Torres, Edgardo, Margarita M. González-Pérez, and Clemente Díaz-Pérez. 2021. 'Barriers and Facilitators to the Participation of Subjects in Clinical Trials: An Overview of Reviews'. *Contemporary Clinical Trials Communications* 23 (September): 100829. <https://doi.org/10.1016/J.CONCTC.2021.100829>.

Roelcke, Volker. 2004. 'Nazi Medicine and Research on Human Beings'. *Lancet* 364 (Suppl. 1): 6–7. <https://doi.org/10.1016/S0140-6736(04)17619-8>.

Rogers, Richard Lee, and Nicolette Powe. 2022. 'COVID-19 Information Sources and Misinformation by Faith Community'. *Inquiry: A Journal of Medical Care Organization, Provision and Financing* 59 (January): 004695802210813. <https://doi.org/10.1177/00469580221081388>.

Rottenburg, Richard. 2009. 'Social and Public Experiments and New Figurations of Science and Politics in Postcolonial Africa1'. *Postcolonial Studies* 12 (4): 423–40. <https://doi.org/10.1080/13688790903350666>.

Sahastrabuddhe, Sushant, and Tarun Saluja. 2019. 'Overview of the Typhoid Conjugate Vaccine Pipeline: Current Status and Future Plans'. *Clinical Infectious Diseases* 68 (Suppl 1): S22. <https://doi.org/10.1093/CID/CIY884>.

Sathian, Brijesh, Mohammad Asim, Indrajit Banerjee, Ana Beatriz Pizarro, Bedanta Roy, Edwin R. van Teijlingen, Israel Júnior Borges do Nascimento, and Hanadi Khamis Alhamad. 2020. 'Impact of COVID-19 on Clinical Trials and Clinical Research: A Systematic Review'. *Nepal Journal of Epidemiology* 10 (3): 878. <https://doi.org/10.3126/NJE.V10I3.31622>.

Schmid, Philipp, and Cornelia Betsch. 2019. 'Effective Strategies for Rebutting Science Denialism in Public Discussions'. *Nature Human Behaviour* 3 (9): 931–9. <https://doi.org/10.1038/s41562-019-0632-4>.

Scott, Pam, Evelleen Richards, and Brian Martin. 1990. 'Captives of Controversy: The Myth of the Neutral Social Researcher in Contemporary Scientific Controversies'. *Science, Technology, & Human Values* 15 (4): 474–94. <https://doi.org/10.1177/016224399001500406>.

Scoy, Lauren Jodi Van, Bethany Snyder, Erin L. Miller, Olubukola Toyobo, Ashmita Grewel, Giang Ha, Sarah Gillespie, et al. 2021. 'Public Anxiety and Distrust

Due to Perceived Politicization and Media Sensationalism during Early COVID-19 Media Messaging'. *Journal of Communication in Healthcare* 14 (3): 193–205. <https://doi.org/10.1080/17538068.2021.1953934>.

Seither, Ranee, Kayla Calhoun, Erica J. Street, Jenelle Mellerson, Cynthia L. Knighton, Ashley Tippins, and J. Michael Underwood. 2019. 'Vaccination Coverage for Selected Vaccines, Exemption Rates, and Provisional Enrollment among Children in Kindergarten – United States, 2016–17 School Year'. *MMWR. Morbidity and Mortality Weekly Report* 66 (40): 1073–80. <https://doi.org/10.15585/MMWR.MM6640A3>.

Sharma, Sanchita. 2019. 'Vaccines Saves Lives, Ignorance Jeopardises Them'. *Hindustan Times*. February 10. <https://www.hindustantimes.com/fitness/vaccines-saves-lives-ignorance-jeopardises-them/story-YygCYbOEDZS45AxZZfvZHJ.html>.

Shiffman, Jeremy. 2009. 'A Social Explanation for the Rise and Fall of Global Health Issues'. *Bulletin of the World Health Organization* 87 (8): 608–13. <https://www.ncbi.nlm.nih.gov/pmc/articles/PMC2733265/>.

Silver, Ira. 1997. 'Constructing "Social Change" through Philanthropy: Boundary Framing and the Articulation of Vocabularies of Motives for Social Movement Participation'. *Sociological Inquiry* 67 (4): 488–503. <https://doi.org/10.1111/j.1475-682X.1997.tb00449.x>.

Sisson, Paul. 2016. 'Lawyers Pull San Diego Lawsuit against California's Controversial Vaccination Law'. *San Diego Union-Tribune*. October 8. <http://www.sandiegouniontribune.com/news/health/sdut-vaccine-lawsuit-sd-pulled-2016sep01-story.html>.

Smallwood, Christine. 2008. 'Back Talk: Paul Offit'. *Nation*. November 3. <https://www.thenation.com/article/archive/back-talk-paul-offit/>.

Smith, Michael J., and Gary S. Marshall. 2010. 'Navigating Parental Vaccine Hesitancy'. *Pediatric Annals* 39 (8): 476–82 <https://doi.org/10.3928/00904481-20100726-05>.

Snape, Matthew D., and Andrew J. Pollard. 2005. 'Meningococcal Polysaccharide–Protein Conjugate Vaccines'. *Lancet Infectious Diseases* 5 (1): 21–30. <https://doi.org/10.1016/S1473-3099(04)01251-4>.

Spier, Ray E. 2001. 'Perception of Risk of Vaccine Adverse Events: A Historical Perspective'. *Vaccine* 20 (October): S78–84. <https://doi.org/10.1016/S0264-410X(01)00306-1>.

Sridhar, Devi, and Rajaie Batniji. 2008. 'Misfinancing Global Health: A Case for Transparency in Disbursements and Decision Making'. *Lancet* 372 (9644): 1185–91. <https://doi.org/10.1016/S0140-6736(08)61485-3>.

Sussex Health & Care Partnership. 2021. 'Covid-19 Vaccination Champions'. <https://assets.publishing.service.gov.uk/gohttps://web.archive.org/web/20220703213446/https://www.sussexhealthandcare.uk/get-involved/covid-19-vaccination-champions/vernment/uploads/system/uploads/attachment_data/file/1011854/A_rapid_scoping_review_of_community_champion_approaches_for_the_pandemic_response_and_recovery_V8.pdf>

Swain, Kelley. 2017. 'The Penicillin Girls (and Guys)'. *Lancet* 389 (10078): 1507. <https://doi.org/10.1016/S0140-6736(17)30957-1>.

Swan, Rita. 2020. 'Faith-Based Medical Neglect: For Providers and Policymakers'. *Journal of Child & Adolescent Trauma* 13 (3): 343. <https://doi.org/10.1007/S40653-020-00323-Z>.

Take on Typhoid. 2011. '10 Years after Typhoid Genome Sequenced – What Is Being Done to Control Typhoid Fever?' <https://www.coalitionagainsttyphoid.org/10-years-after-typhoid-genome-sequenced-what-is-being-done-to-control-typhoid-fever/>.

Tam, Ng Uyen Thanh, Le Thi Bich Thoa, Nguyen Phuoc Long, Nguyen Thi Huyen Trang, Kenji Hirayama, Juntra Karbwang, and Nguyen Tien Huy. 2015. 'Participants' Understanding of Informed Consent in Clinical Trials over Three Decades: Systematic Review and Meta-Analysis'. *Bulletin of the World Health Organization* 93 (3): 186. <https://doi.org/10.2471/BLT.14.141390>.

Tavares, Tânia D., Joana C. Antunes, Jorge Padrão, Ana I. Ribeiro, Andrea Zille, M. Teresa P. Amorim, Fernando Ferreira, and Helena P. Felgueiras. 2020. 'Activity of Specialized Biomolecules against Gram-Positive and Gram-Negative Bacteria'. *Antibiotics* 9 (6): 314. <https://doi.org/10.3390/ANTIBIOTICS9060314>.

Tengbeh, Angus Fayia, Luisa Enria, Elizabeth Smout, Thomas Mooney, Mike Callaghan, David Ishola, Bailah Leigh, et al. 2018. ' "We Are the Heroes Because We Are Ready to Die for This Country": Participants' Decision-Making and Grounded Ethics in an Ebola Vaccine Clinical Trial'. *Social Science & Medicine* 203 (April): 35–42. <https://doi.org/10.1016/J.SOCSCIMED.2018.03.008>.

Thomas, Ryan J., Edson C. Tandoc, and Amanda Hinnant. 2017. 'False Balance in Public Health Reporting? Michele Bachmann, the HPV Vaccine, and "Mental Retardation" '. *Health Communication* 32 (2): 152–60. <https://doi.org/10.1080/10410236.2015.1110006>.

Thomas, Tonia M., Susanne H. Hodgson, Katherine Emary, Maia Patrick-Smith, Rebecca Te Water Naude, Arabella S.V. Stuart, John Henry, et al. 2023. 'The Collective Voice of Early Phase COVID-19 Vaccine Trial Participants: Insights for Improving Confidence in Novel Vaccines'. *Human Vaccines & Immunotherapeutics* 19 (1): 2203023. <https://doi.org/10.1080/21645515.2023.2203023>.

Thompson, Alex, Holly Otterbein, and Alice Miranda Ollstein. 2020. 'Anti-Vaxx Politicians under Fire as Coronavirus Spreads'. *Politico*. <https://www.politico.com/news/2020/03/21/anti-vaccine-coronavirus-137446>.

Thorp, Holden. H. 2020. 'Trump's Rhetoric Will Make the Pandemic Worse: Words Are Now a Matter of Life and Death'. *Guardian*. <https://www.theguardian.com/global/commentisfree/2020/mar/13/trump-coronavirus-antivaxxer-vaccine>.

Tomes, Nancy. 2002. 'Epidemic Entertainments: Disease and Popular Culture in Early-Twentieth-Century America'. *American Literary History* 14 (4): 625–52. <https://doi.org/10.1093/ALH/14.4.625>.

Törnberg, Petter. 2018. 'Echo Chambers and Viral Misinformation: Modeling Fake News as Complex Contagion'. *PLOS ONE* 13 (9): e0203958. <https://doi.org/10.1371/JOURNAL.PONE.0203958>.

Tripathi, Ashutosh. 2017. 'Vaccination Drive Extended after Hitting a Wall in Muslim Pockets'. *News18.Com*. February 25. <https://www.news18.com/news/india/vaccination-drive-extended-as-campaign-hits-propaganda-wall-in-mus lim-pockets-1352897.html>.

Turner, Paul J., Heidi Larson, Eve Dubé, and Allison Fisher. 2021. 'Vaccine Hesitancy: Drivers and How the Allergy Community Can Help'. *Journal of Allergy and Clinical Immunology: In Practice* 9 (10): 3568–74. <https://doi.org/10.1016/J.JAIP.2021.06.035>.

Typhoid Swallowers. 2020. 'Typhoidland Project'. Accessed 10 July 2024. <https://www.youtube.com/watch?v=fuYcgcBMfjQ>.

Vaccinate California. n.d. 'Vaccinate California Webpage'. Accessed 16 July 2017. <http://vaccinatecalifornia.org/>.

Vaccine Knowledge. n.d. 'Vaccine Knowledge'. Accessed 10 July 2024. <http://vk.ovg.ox.ac.uk/>.

Vaidya, Sunil R., Madhukar B. Kamble, Deepika T. Chowdhury, and Neelakshi S. Kumbhar. 2016. 'Measles Rubella Outbreaks in Maharashtra State, India'. *Indian Journal of Medical Research* 143 (2): 227. <https://doi.org/10.4103/0971-5916.180214>.

Valent, Peter, Bernd Groner, Udo Schumacher, Giulio Superti-Furga, Meinrad Busslinger, Robert Kralovics, Christoph Zielinski, et al. 2016. 'Paul Ehrlich (1854–1915) and His Contributions to the Foundation and Birth of Translational Medicine'. *Journal of Innate Immunity* 8 (2): 111–20. <https://doi.org/10.1159/000443526>.

Vanderslott, Samantha, Andrew Pollard, and Tonia Thomas. 2020. 'Coronavirus Vaccine: Here Are the Steps It Will Need to Go through during Development'. *Conversation*. <https://theconversation.com/coronavirus-vaccine-here-are-the-steps-it-will-need-to-go-through-during-development-134726>.

Vanderslott, Samantha. 2017. 'Despite Scepticism, Europe Has High Vaccination Rates – but It Shouldn't Be Complacent'. *Conversation*. <https://theconversation.com/despite-scepticism-europe-has-high-vaccination-rates-but-it-shouldnt-be-complacent-75169>.

Vanderslott, Samantha. 2018. 'Anti-Vaxxer Effect on Vaccination Rates Is Exaggerated'. *Conversation*. <https://theconversation.com/anti-vaxxer-effect-on-vaccination-rates-is-exaggerated-92630>.

Vanderslott, Samantha. 2019. 'Exploring the Meaning of Pro-Vaccine Activism across Two Countries'. *Social Science & Medicine* 222 (February): 59–66. <https://doi.org/10.1016/J.SOCSCIMED.2018.12.033>.

Vanderslott, Samantha. 2021. 'Greece to Make COVID Vaccines Mandatory for Over-60s, but Do Vaccine Mandates Work?' *Conversation*, 1 December. <https://theconversation.com/greece-to-make-covid-vaccines-mandatory-for-over-60s-but-do-vaccine-mandates-work-172672>.

Vanderslott, Samantha, and Tatjana Marks. 2021. 'Charting Mandatory Childhood Vaccination Policies Worldwide'. *Vaccine*, June. <https://doi.org/10.1016/J.VACCINE.2021.04.065>.

Vanderslott, Samantha, Maile T. Phillips, Virginia E. Pitzer, and Claas Kirchhelle. 2019. 'Water and Filth: Reevaluating the First Era of Sanitary Typhoid Intervention (1840–1940)'. *Clinical Infectious Diseases* 69 (suppl. 5): S377–84. <https://doi.org/10.1093/cid/ciz610>.

Vanderslott, Samantha, Katherine Emary, Rebecca Te, Water Naude, Marcus English, Tonia Thomas, Maia Patrick-Smith, et al. 2021. 'Vaccine Nationalism and Internationalism: Perspectives of COVID-19 Vaccine Trial Participants in the United Kingdom'. *BMJ Global Health* 6 (10): e006305. <https://doi.org/10.1136/BMJGH-2021-006305>.

Vanderslott, Samantha, Alexandra Palmer, Tonia Thomas, Beth Greenhough, Arabella Stuart, John A. Henry, Marcus English, et al. 2021. 'Co-producing Human and Animal Experimental Subjects: Exploring the Views of UK COVID-19 Vaccine Trial Participants on Animal Testing'. *Science, Technology, & Human Values*, 48(4): 909–37. <https://doi.org/10.1177/01622439211057084>.

Vanderslott, Samantha, Manya Van Ryneveld, Mark Marchant, Shelley Lees, Sylvie Kwedi Nolna, and Vicki Marsh. 2021. 'How Can Community Engagement in Health Research Be Strengthened for Infectious Disease Outbreaks in Sub-Saharan Africa? A Scoping Review of the Literature'. *BMC Public Health* 21 (1): 633. <https://doi.org/10.1186/s12889-021-10348-0>.

Vanderslott, Samantha, Kate Joynes-Burgess, Seilesh Kadambari, Emma O'Dwyer, Lailah Alidu, Emma O'Dwyer, Tushna Vandrevala, 2024. 'Examining the role of community champions to promote vaccine uptake in under-served communities in the United Kingdom: Lessons from the COVID-19 pandemic'. *SSM-Qualitative Research in Health*. 5:100436. pp. 1–10. <https://doi.org/10.1016/j.ssmqr.2024.100436>.

Vanderslott, Samantha, Luisa Enria, Alex Bowmer, Alex Bowmer, Abass Kamara, and Shelley Lees. 2022. 'Attributing Public Ignorance in Vaccination Narratives'. *Social Science & Medicine*, 307: 115152. <https://doi.org/10.1016/J.SOCSCIMED.2022.115152>.

Velmet, Aro. 2020. 'Pasteur's Empire'. *Pasteur's Empire*, Oxford: Oxford University Press. <https://doi.org/10.1093/OSO/9780190072827.001.0001>.

Venkatraman, A., N. Garg, and N. Kumar. 2015. 'Greater freedom of speech on Web 2.0 correlates with dominance of views linking vaccines to autism'. *Vaccine*, 33 (12): 1422–1425. <https://doi.org/10.1016/j.vaccine.2015.01.078>

Verger, Pierre, Lisa Fressard, Fanny Collange, Arnaud Gautier, Christine Jestin, Odile Launay, Jocelyn Raude, Céline Pulcini, and Patrick Peretti-Watel. 2015. 'Vaccine Hesitancy among General Practitioners and Its Determinants during Controversies: A National Cross-Sectional Survey in France'. *EBioMedicine* 2 (8): 891–7. <https://doi.org/10.1016/j.ebiom.2015.06.018>.

Verger, Pierre, Elisabeth Botelho-Nevers, Amanda Garrison, Dominique Gagnon, Arnaud Gagneur, Amandine Gagneux-Brunon, and Eve Dubé. 2022. 'Vaccine Hesitancy in Health-Care Providers in Western Countries: A Narrative Review'. *Expert Review of Vaccines* 21 (7): 909–27. <https://doi.org/10.1080/14760584.2022.2056026>.

Vignaud, Laurent-Henri, and Françoise Salvadori. 2019. *ANTIVAX. La Résistance Aux Vaccins Du XVIIIe Siècle à Nos Jours*, Vendémiaire. <https://hal-univ-bourgogne.archives-ouvertes.fr/hal-01984504>.

Volokh, Eugene. 2015. 'Family Court Gives Pro-vaccination Father Decisionmaking Authority over Children's Medical Care'. *Washington Post*. <https://www.washingtonpost.com/news/volokh-conspiracy/wp/2015/04/06/family-court-gives-pro-vaccination-father-decisionmaking-authority-over-childrens-medical-care/>.

Wang, Eileen, Yelena Baras, and Alison M. Buttenheim. 2015. '"Everybody Just Wants to Do What's Best for Their Child": Understanding How Pro-vaccine Parents Can Support a Culture of Vaccine Hesitancy'. *Vaccine* 33 (48): 6703–9. <https://doi.org/10.1016/J.VACCINE.2015.10.090>.

Ward, Jeremy K. 2016. 'Rethinking the Antivaccine Movement Concept: A Case Study of Public Criticism of the Swine Flu Vaccine's Safety in France'. *Social Science & Medicine* 159 (June): 48–57. <https://doi.org/10.1016/J.SOCSCIMED.2016.05.003>.

Warne, Chris. 2013. 'Stroud Charity Takes Its Campaign for a New Meningitis Vaccine to Downing Street'. *Stroud News and Journal*. <https://www.stroudnewsandjournal.co.uk/news/10772272.stroud-charity-takes-its-campaign-for-a-new-meningitis-vaccine-to-downing-street/>.

Washer, Peter. 2010. 'Emerging Infectious Diseases and Society'. *Emerging Infectious Diseases and Society*, 1–191. New York: Palgrave Macmillan.

Watson, Christopher. 2020. 'House of Commons Trends: E-Petitions'. *House of Commons Library*. <https://commonslibrary.parliament.uk/house-of-commons-trends-e-petitions/>.

Way, Fran. 2020. 'Oxford University Want Volunteers for Coronavirus Vaccine'. *Oxford Mail*. <https://www.oxfordmail.co.uk/news/18340268.oxford-university-want-volunteers-coronavirus-vaccine/>.

Weber Shandwick. 2018. 'The Great American Search for Healthcare Information'. <https://www.webershandwick.com/news/the-great-american-search-for-healthcare-information/>.

Weindling, Paul. 2001. 'The Origins of Informed Consent: The International Scientific Commission on Medical War Crimes, and the Nuremburg Code'. *Bulletin of the History of Medicine* 75 (1): 37–71. <https://doi.org/10.1353/BHM.2001.0049>.

Wellcome Global Monitor. 2018. 'How Does the World Feel about Science and Health'. *Wellcome Trust*. <https://wellcome.org/reports/wellcome-global-monitor/2018>.

Wentzell, Emily, and Ana-Monica Racila. 2021. 'Collective Care Amid US Individualism through COVID-19 Vaccine Trial Participation'. *Medical Anthropology*, November, 1–15. <https://doi.org/10.1080/01459740.2021.1998041>.

Whatmore, Sarah J., and Catharina Landström. 2011. 'Flood Apprentices: An Exercise in Making Things Public'. *Economy and Society* 40 (4): 582–610. <https://doi.org/10.1080/03085147.2011.602540>.

Whatthefolly. 2015. 'Transcript: Mother & Pro-Vaccination Advocate Leah Russin's Testimony on SB 277 before the Senate Judiciary Committee – April 28, 2015'. <http://www.whatthefolly.com/2015/04/30/transcript-mother-pro-vaccination-advocate-leah-russins-testimony-on-sb-277-before-the-senate-judiciary-committee-april-28-2015/>.

WHO. 2015. 'Zoonoses'. Accessed 3 April 2024. <https://www.who.int/news-room/fact-sheets/detail/zoonoses>.

WHO. 2017. 'Global Vaccine Action Plan 2011–2020'. <https://www.who.int/immunization/global_vaccine_action_plan/GVAP_doc_2011_2020/en/>.

WHO. 2019a. 'Against All Odds, India Set to Make History yet Again'. <https://www.who.int/india/news/feature-stories/detail/against-all-odds-india-set-to-make-history-yet-again>.

WHO. 2019b. 'Ten Threats to Global Health in 2019'. <https://www.who.int/news-room/spotlight/ten-threats-to-global-health-in-2019>.

WHO. 2020. 'Managing the COVID-19 Infodemic: Promoting Healthy Behaviours and Mitigating the Harm from Misinformation and Disinformation'. Joint Statement by WHO, UN, UNICEF, UNDP, UNESCO, UNAIDS, ITU, UN Global Pulse, and IFRC. <https://www.who.int/news/item/23-09-2020-managing-the-covid-19-infodemic-promoting-healthy-behaviours-and-mitigating-the-harm-from-misinformation-and-disinformation>.

WHO. 2022. 'Moving towards the Measles and Rubella Elimination Goal in India'. <https://www.who.int/india/news/feature-stories/detail/moving-towards-the-measles-and-rubella-elimination-goal-in-india>.

WHO. n.d. 'Meningitis'. Accessed 31 July 2022. <https://www.who.int/news-room/fact-sheets/detail/meningitis>.

WHO. n.d. 'Typhoid'. Accessed 26 June 2023. <https://www.who.int/health-topics/typhoid#tab=tab_1>.

Williams, Naomi. 1994. 'The Implementation of Compulsory Health Legislation: Infant Smallpox Vaccination in England and Wales, 1840–1890'. *Journal of Historical Geography* 20 (4): 396–412. <https://doi.org/10.1006/JHGE.1994.1031>.

Wilson, John. 1973. *Introduction to Social Movements*. New York: Basic Books.

Wise, Jacqui. 1999. 'UK Introduces New Meningitis C Vaccine'. *BMJ* 319 (7205): 278. <https://doi.org/10.1136/BMJ.319.7205.278>.

Woolston, Chris. 2020. '"I've Never Worked Harder": The Race to Develop a COVID-19 Vaccine'. *Nature* 587 (7833): 322. <https://doi.org/10.1038/D41586-020-03139-X>.

Yao, Bin, Li Zhu, Qi Jiang, and H. Xia. 2013. 'Safety Monitoring in Clinical Trials'. *Pharmaceutics* 5 (4): 94–106. <https://doi.org/10.3390/pharmaceutics5010094>.

Yaqub, Ohid, Sophie Castle-Clarke, Nick Sevdalis, and Joanna Chataway. 2014. 'Attitudes to Vaccination: A Critical Review'. *Social Science & Medicine* 112: 1–11. <https://doi.org/10.1016/j.socscimed.2014.04.018>.

Zarei, Adi Essam, Hussein A. Almehdar, and Elrashdy M. Redwan. 2016. 'Hib Vaccines: Past, Present, and Future Perspectives'. *Journal of Immunology Research*. (1): 7203587. <https://doi.org/10.1155/2016/7203587>.

Zarocostas, John. 2020. 'How to Fight an Infodemic'. *Lancet* 395 (10225): 676. <https://doi.org/10.1016/S0140-6736(20)30461-X>.

Zimmer, Carl. 2020. '3 Covid-19 Trials Have Been Paused for Safety: That's a Good Thing'. *New York Times*. <https://www.nytimes.com/2020/10/14/health/covid-clinical-trials.html>.

Zinn, Jens O. 2008. 'Heading into the Unknown: Everyday Strategies for Managing Risk and Uncertainty'. *Health, Risk & Society* 10 (5): 439–50. <https://doi.org/10.1080/13698570802380891>.

Index

Medical Humanities: Criticism and Creativity

Series Editors: Maria Vaccarella, MA, PhD, Senior Lecturer in Medical Humanities, University of Bristol and Kimberly R. Myers, MA, PhD, Professor of Humanities and Medicine, Penn State College of Medicine

This series showcases innovative research, creativity and pedagogy in the interdisciplinary field of medical humanities. Books in the series explore the complexities of human bodies, minds, illness, and wellbeing through analytical frameworks derived from humanistic disciplines and clinical practice. The series publishes a range of materials, including monographs and edited collections on scholarly approaches to medical issues in culture; creative works (accompanied by analytical and educational materials) that engage with medical humanities themes; and critical, engaged or radical pedagogies on focused topics for learners in the medical and health humanities.

Medical Humanities: Criticism and Creativity is intended to provide an informative exchange across disciplines, encouraging theoretical and personal reflections on the condition of the human mind/body and contributing to debates on health-related issues from a broad range of perspectives. The series also invites research that opens up critical conversations on being human at the intersection of other forms of humanistic knowledge, such as environmental and digital humanities. We are especially interested in collaborations between academics in the humanities and healthcare professionals.

All book proposals and manuscripts undergo rigorous peer review prior to acceptance and publication.

(Oregon Health and Science University), Barry Saunders (University of North Carolina School of Medicine), Johanna Shapiro (University of California, Irvine, School of Medicine), Marina Tsaplina (The Betes Organization), Craigan Usher (Oregon Health and Science University), Neil Vickers (King's College London), Martin Willis (Cardiff University), Charlotte Wu (Boston University School of Medicine)

Kimberly R. Myers (ed.), *Breast Cancer Inside Out: Bodies, Biographies & Beliefs*.
2021. ISBN 978-1-78874-733-2.

Lisbeth Frølunde, Louise Phillips and Maria Bee Christensen-Strynø, *Moving along: A co-produced graphic novel about Parkinson's dance.*
2023. ISBN 978-1-80079-934-9.

Darian Goldin Stahl, *Embodied Books: Experiencing the Health Humanities through Artists' Books.*
2024. ISBN 978-1-80079-816-8.

Samantha Vanderslott, *Pro-vax: Supporting Vaccines through Activism, Petitions, and Trials*.
2025. ISBN 978-1-80079-470-2